Portal Design
in Radiation
Therapy
3rd Edition

Portal Design in Radiation Therapy
3rd Edition

Anne Marie Vann, M.Ed., C.M.D, R.T.(R)(T)
Byron G. Dasher, M.D.
Nancy H. Wiggers, M.D.
Sharon K. Chestnut, M.Ed., C.M.D, R.T.(T)

Illustrations by Kirah L. Van Sickle, M.S.M.I.
Reviewed by Patrick S. Markwalter, M.D.

Phoenix Printing

Anne Marie Vann, M.Ed, C.M.D., R.T.T.
Past Program Director, Radiation Therapy/Medical Dosimetry
Medical College of Georgia
Augusta, Georgia

Byron G. Dasher, M.D.
Radiation Oncology Associates
Georgia Radiation Therapy Center
Augusta, Georgia

Nancy H. Wiggers, M.D.
Northside Radiation Oncology Care
Northside Hospital
Atlanta, Georgia

Sharon K. Chestnut, M.Ed., C.M.D., R.T.T.
Assistant Professor
Radiation Therapy
Georgia Regents University
Augusta, Georgia

Patrick S. Markwalter, M.D.
Fellow of Musculoskeletal Radiology
Forsyth Radiological Associates
Winston Salem, North Carolina

© 2013 DWV Enterprises

Printed in the United States of America
1st Edition: 1994
2nd Edition: 2006
3rd Edition: 2013

Library of Congress Catalog Card Number: 94-7251

Phoenix Printing
601 11th Street
Augusta, GA 30901

Preface

It was the intent of the authors to design a textbook that can be used by radiation therapists and oncologists as a quick reference when simulating treatment portals. With the realization that a portal must be designed for each individual patient, the authors have described typical treatment portals to provide a guideline for simulation and treatment. For the unusual circumstances, the anatomy and primary routes of spread are discussed to allow the reader to tailor treatment portals based on the anatomical facts. This text includes only those sites where radiation is traditionally indicated in the patient's management.

Disclaimer

The authors realize the normal tissue complication probability is dependent on a variety of factors including, but not limited to: dose uniformity within the irradiated volume, variation of radiosensitivity within the irradiated tissue itself, dose fraction, volume and non-radiation factors including patient health status and chemotherapy. We have chosen to list the traditional normal tissue tolerance doses as published by Emami, et al. (1991) and the updated QUANTEC (Qualitative Analysis of Normal Tissue Effects in the Clinic) guidelines published by L. B. Marks, et al. in the International Journal of Radiation Oncology Biology and Physics 2010.

VI

Table of Contents

VIII

x

Chapter 1

Head and Neck Cancer

TREATMENT OF THE NECK

Treatment of the lymph nodes in primary head and neck cancers depends on many factors:

1) the site of primary disease (nasopharyngeal and pyriform sinus have a rich capillary lymphatic network as opposed to paranasal sinus, middle ear and vocal cords that have no capillary lymphatics)
2) the extent of primary disease (lymph node metastases increase with depth of invasion and extension into sites with rich capillary lymphatics)
3) size of the primary tumor (except for tumors of the nasopharynx and pyriform sinus which metastasize independent of tumor size)
4) cell type and differentiation (the more poorly differentiated, the greater the risk of lymph node metastases)
5) lymphatic vascular space invasion of the tumor
6) the clinical, or present nodal status of the patient

Anatomy

The first echelon of lymph nodes are usually included in the treatment portal encompassing the primary tumor. The supraclavicular and lower neck is generally treated when there is macroscopic or a risk for microscopic disease in this area. The lymph node regions that will be discussed in this chapter are diagramed in Figs. 1.1 and 1.2.

Note that there are no posterior cervical nodes located behind the spinous processes.

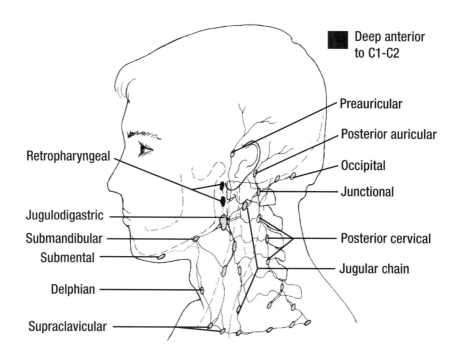

Fig. 1.1 Lymph Nodes of the Head and Neck

Lymph nodes in the neck have been divided into 7 levels as illustrated below

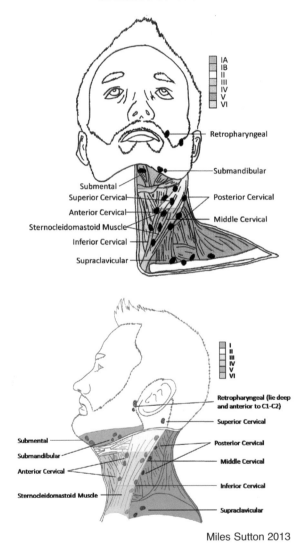

Miles Sutton 2013

Fig 1.2

The retropharyngeal nodes are located behind the pharynx and extend from the base of the skull down to the hyoid bone

Treatment

For patients with No or N1 disease, ipsilateral high risk nodal groups may be selectively irradiated. For tumors with a high incidence of nodal spread (e.g., nasopharynx) and tumors staged N2a or greater, bilateral irradiation of all neck node levels is recommended. Patients with prior neck surgery may have rerouting of the lymphatics; and therefore all neck levels should be irradiated.

Technical Aspects of Radiation Therapy

Intensity Modulated Radiation Therapy (IMRT) has led to significant advancements when treating head and neck cancers. IMRT allows for conformal radiation delivery to image based targets while sparing critical structures by using arcs or multiple non-opposed beams that intersect within the target volume and multi-leaf collimation (MLC). Understanding anatomy including areas at risk for disease and toxicity and dose tolerance of critical structures is important. Definitions for treatment planning:

GTV Gross tumor volume
(generally the volume discernible from imaging)

CTV Clinical target volume - expansion of the GTV for uncertainty about tumor extent (microscopic extension, contouring variability) - does not typically cross natural interfaces, i.e. from soft tissue into bone unless invasion is suspected

PTV Planning target volume- expansion of the CTV for geometric uncertainty (setup variation, organ motion) - while GTV and PTV should not exit patient, PTV is GEOMETRIC not anatomic

ITV Internal target volume- expansion of CTV for internal (e.g. breathing) movement

OAR Organ at risk

PRV Planning organ at risk volume- expansion of OAR for movement

The GTVs and CTVs are drawn on the axial CT images. MRI, CT, and PET scans can be fused with the treatment planning CT to better delineate these structures. A uniform expansion is then performed to accommodate set up uncertainties (3-5 mm).

IMRT is able to conform the dose to the target (GTV) and spare critical surrounding structures (OAR's), such as the spinal cord, larynx and parotid glands in the head and neck. IMRT also enables the radiation oncologist to prescribe a total dose to the tumor volume and the surrounding lymph nodes. In this case each dose region would be delineated with a PTV. This method of treatment is known as a simultaneous integrated boost (SIB) and is illustrated in Fig 1.3:

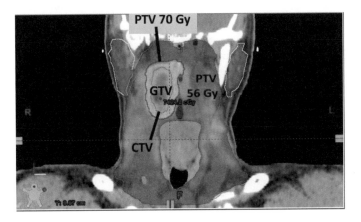

Fig 1.3

Treatment

The patient is generally positioned supine for all head and neck treatment. An aquaplast mask or appropriate immobilization device is used. The shoulders are depressed and immobilized so that beams may clear the shoulders. If lower cervical neck nodes must be treated, the treatment couch can be angled to avoid beam entrance into the shoulders.

For tumors of the oral cavity, oropharynx, and nasopharynx the laryngeal structures can be spared with blocking when the primary lesion does not extend beyond the thyroid notch. The tracheal stoma should be electively treated in patients who have had an emergency tracheostomy, who exhibit subglottic extension, close or positive margins, or involvement of soft tissues of the neck. An IMRT technique is the treatment of choice for the majority of head and neck cases. However, a traditional three field setup may be required based upon the patient's condition, tumor location and extent, or physician preference. Two opposed lateral fields encompassing the primary tumor can be abutted to an anterior neck node field. This 3 field arrangement is generally accomplished using a half beam technique as illustrated below:

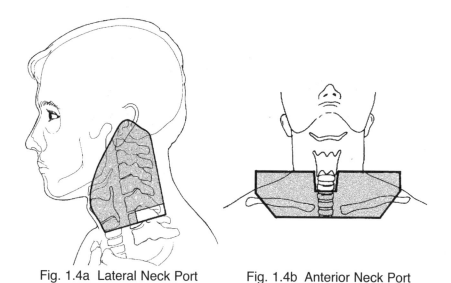

Fig. 1.4a Lateral Neck Port   Fig. 1.4b Anterior Neck Port

Most centers use a half-beam block at the junction of the anterior and lateral ports to prevent overlap of the fields. If the central ray is not utilized at the match line, then the collimator must be angled on the lateral fields to match the beam divergence from the anterior field. Spinal cord blocks should always be added in either the anterior or lateral fields to assure that the beams did not overlap in this area. The lateral fields are usually reduced off of the spinal cord at 45 Gy. When the posterior cervical nodes are at risk, they may be boosted with electrons to increase the dose to the nodes while sparing the spinal cord from additional radiation.

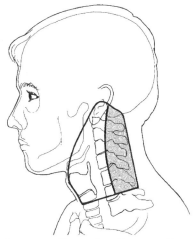

Fig. 1.5a Posterior Electron Port

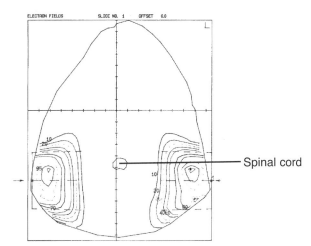

Fig. 1.5b 9 MeV Electron Dose Distribution

ORAL CAVITY

Oral cavity tumors account for less than 5% of all carcinomas in the United States. Over 80% of oral cavity tumors are keratinizing squamous cell carcinomas. Non-keratinizing squamous cell and minor salivary gland tumors are also found in this area. Basal cell carcinomas may arise from the skin of the lip.

Carcinoma of the lip constitutes about 45%, the oral tongue 17%, and the floor of the mouth 12%, of all oral cavity malignancies. Patients that smoke, consume alcohol, or who have poor dental hygiene, are at an increased risk of intraoral cancer. Carcinomas of the lip are related to sunlight exposure.

Anatomy

The oral cavity consists of the lip, floor of mouth, oral tongue (anterior two-thirds), buccal mucosa, upper and lower gingiva, hard palate, and retromolar trigone.

The mylohyoid muscle forms the floor of the oral cavity. The roof of the oral cavity is the hard palate. Anteriorly the oral cavity extends to the skin-vermillion junction. Posteriorly, the oral cavity extends to the retromolar trigone (which is a triangular area of mucosa which covers the mandible, posterior to the last molar tooth), and the posterior oral tongue, which is separated from the base of the tongue by the circumvallate papillae.

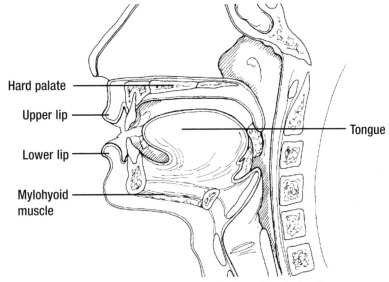

Fig. 1.6 Boundaries of the Oral Cavity

CARCINOMA OF THE LIP

Routes of Spread

Squamous cell carcinomas of the lip most commonly arise from the lower lip and spread by direct invasion. Lip carcinomas present with lymph node metastases 5-10% of the time. The lip drains to lymph nodes in the submental, submaxillary and jugulodigastric regions. Lymph node involvement increases with large lesions, poorly differentiated tumors, spread to the wet mucosal surfaces, invasion of the dermis, or recurrent disease.

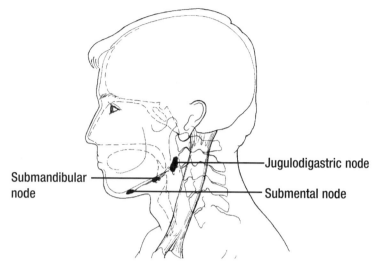

Fig. 1.7 Lymph Drainage of the Lip

Treatment

Carcinoma in-situ and early lesions of the lip (less than 0.5-1.5 cm) may be treated with surgical excision alone. Radiation therapy is used for commissure lesions, or lesions that would create a large surgical or functional defect (upper lip lesion or greater than 1.5 cm of the lower lip). Advanced lesions with bone or neural invasion require resection and postoperative radiation.

Technical Aspects of Radiation Therapy

The radiation portal should include the primary lesion with a 2 cm margin. A shield made of lead and a bolus material to absorb backscatter, should be placed under the lip to block the alveolar process and gums. Elective neck treatment may be withheld since neck failures from lip cancers have proven to be salvageable.

Dose

Lip treatment can be given with superficial x-rays, electrons, or with brachytherapy.
External beam doses: 60-70 Gy at 2.0 Gy per fraction, depending on the size of the lesion and method of treatment.

FLOOR OF MOUTH AND ORAL TONGUE

Routes of Spread

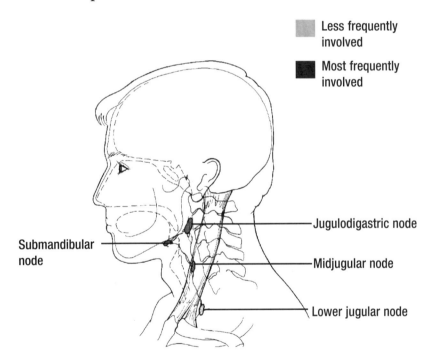

Less frequently involved

Most frequently involved

Jugulodigastric node

Submandibular node

Midjugular node

Lower jugular node

Fig. 1.8 Lymph Drainage for Floor of Mouth

Floor of mouth and oral tongue lesions more commonly present with lymph node metastases with an incidence of 35-40%. The primary nodal drainage is to the jugulodigastric, midjugular, and submaxillary lymph nodes. These are usually midline tumors and therefore bilateral lymph node chains are at risk for disease. These tumors may infiltrate locally to involve underlying muscle, or extend along fibro-fatty planes.

Treatment

Surgery and radiation therapy both have similar cure rates for T1 and T2 (4 cm or less) cancers of the floor of mouth and oral tongue.

Treatment is generally given by external beam which provides treatment to the primary lesion and neck nodes. The intraoral cone or an interstitial implant can be used for small cancers, as definitive treatment or as a boost. The advantage of using the intraoral cone or an interstitial implant is sparing the normal tissues that would otherwise be included in the external beam portal. If the intraoral cone is used in conjunction with external beam, the cone field should be treated before the large lateral fields so that the patient can tolerate manipulation of the mouth before mucositis begins.

Surgery with postoperative radiation is advocated for T3 or T4 tumors (greater than 4 cm or with invasion of adjacent structures), close or positive margins, perineural or lymphatic vascular invasion, or multiple positive nodes.

Technical Aspects of Radiation Therapy

The borders for the lateral fields for floor of mouth or oral tongue include:

Anterior: in front of the mandible (exclude the lower lip if possible)

Posterior: *node negative* - behind vertebral bodies
node positive - behind spinous processes

Superior: 1.5 cm above the tongue

Inferior: thyroid notch

A tongue blade is used to raise the roof of the mouth out of the treatment field.

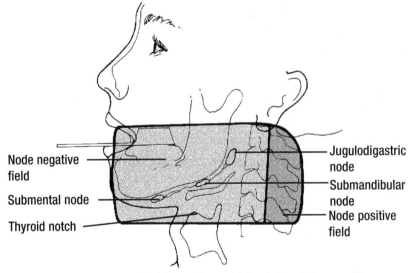

Fig. 1.9 Treatment Field for Floor of Mouth/Oral Tongue Tumor

NOTE: In patients with well-lateralized lesions and clinically negative neck nodes, an ipsilateral anterior neck field is treated. Bilateral neck nodes must be treated for midline tumors, or with patients with positive nodes.

CT ANATOMY

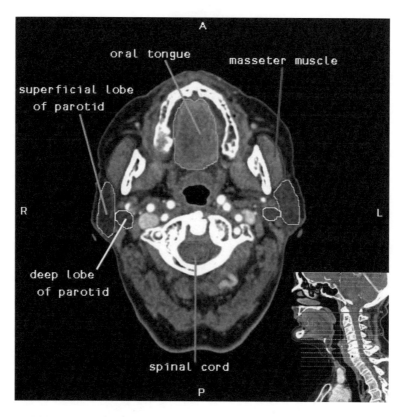

TOLERANCE DOSES

TD5/5 Normal Tissue Tolerances (Gy) 1.8-2.0 Gy/fraction				
Organ	1/3	2/3	3/3	End Point
Parotid	32	32	32	Xerostomia
Spinal Cord	50 (5cm)	50 (10 cm)	47 (20 cm)	Myelitis/Necrosis
Temporomandibular joint & mandible	61	60	60	Marked limitation of the joint function

Note: Qualitative Analysis of Normal Tissue Effects in the Clinic (QUANTEC) data suggests when sparing one parotid the mean dose should not exceed 20 Gy. When both parotid glands are spared, the mean dose to both glands should not exceed 25 Gy.

L.B. Marks, et. al., Use of Normal Tissue Complication Probability in the Clinic, IJROBP, Vol 76, No. 3, Supplement 2010, S10-S19.

OROPHARYNX

Carcinomas of the oropharynx are relatively rare head and neck cancers. 95% of oropharyngeal lesions are squamous cell carcinomas. Lymphomas and lymphoepithelial tumors are rare but can occur in the tonsil and in the base of the tongue. Risk factors include smoking, alcohol consumption, and poor dental hygiene.

Anatomy

The oropharynx includes the base of the tongue, the tonsillar region, (the vallecula is considered part of the tonsillar fossa and pillars), the soft palate, and the portion of the pharyngeal wall between the pharyngoepiglottic fold and the nasopharynx. The oropharynx is bound anteriorly by the circumvallate papillae, and the junction of the hard and soft palate. The oropharynx extends from the highest aspect of the soft palate superiorly to the hyoid bone inferiorly and is bound posteriorly by the posterior pharyngeal wall.

Boundaries of the Orophayrnx

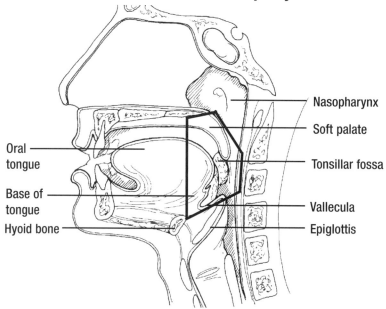

Nasopharynx

Soft palate

Oral tongue

Tonsillar fossa

Base of tongue

Vallecula

Hyoid bone

Epiglottis

Fig. 1.10a

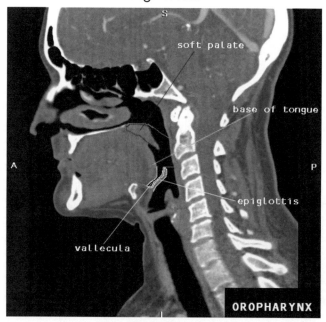

Fig. 1.10b

Routes of Spread

Oropharyngeal tumors spread primarily by direct extension or through the lymphatics. Hematogenous spread can occur with advanced or recurrent tumors. The most common site of hematogenous metastases is the lungs.

The first echelon of lymph node drainage of the oropharyngeal region is to the jugulodigastric and midjugular nodes. The incidence of lymph node involvement, and the risk of bilateral disease, or positive cervical nodes, depends on the location and the size of the primary tumor.

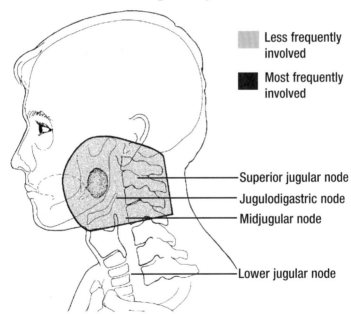

Less frequently involved

Most frequently involved

Superior jugular node
Jugulodigastric node
Midjugular node

Lower jugular node

Fig 1.11 Lymph Drainage of the Oropharynx

Technical Aspects of Radiation Therapy

Radiation therapy is the treatment of choice for early stage oropharyngeal tumors. Large extensive tumors are treated with combined surgery and postoperative radiation.

Radiation therapy alone is often used for inoperable patients and for palliation.

Treatment borders for tumors of the oropharynx:

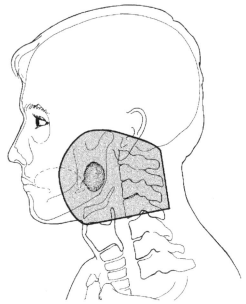

Fig. 1.12 Treatment Borders for Oropharynx Tumor

Anterior: 2 cm anterior to the tumor
Posterior: behind the spinous process (to include the posterior cervical lymph nodes)
Superior: entire jugular chain and above C1 (to include the retropharyngeal lymph nodes)
Inferior: thyroid notch, or to include the supraclavicular area

The supraclavicular and lower jugular lymph nodes can be included with IMRT treatment of the primary, or a separate anterior lower neck field can be abutted to the primary field Treatment of the lower neck is essential because of the high rate of bilateral lymph node metastases even if the neck is clinically negative. Tonsillar lesions which are lateralized may only need ipsilateral neck node treatment.

For tumors of the base of tongue, the final boost field may be administered by interstitial implant (for small anterior-lateral lesions), a submental external beam portal, or a reduced lateral field.

Postoperative treatment is advocated with close or positive margins, multiple positive lymph nodes, extracapsular extension, or elective neck coverage.

CT ANATOMY

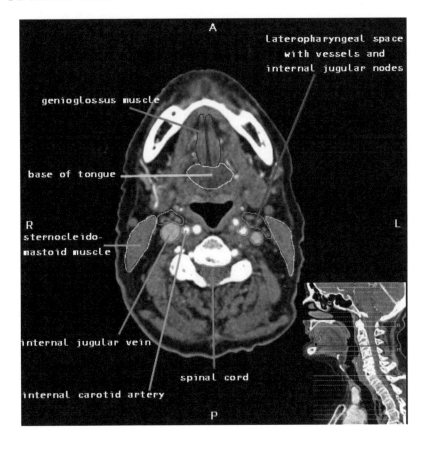

LARYNX

Carcinoma of the larynx is the most common cancer of the head and neck. 65% of laryngeal carcinomas occur in the glottic larynx and 34% occur in the supraglottic larynx. Subglottic carcinomas are rare, comprising only 1% of all glottic cancers.

Laryngeal cancers are more common in men than in women, with a ratio of 5:1. Cigarette smoking is a known etiologic factor for laryngeal cancer. The most common histology is squamous cell. Patients with vocal cord carcinoma commonly present with hoarseness, while supraglottic tumors can cause sore throat and odynophagia.

Anatomy

The larynx is subdivided into three regions: the supraglottis, the glottis, and the subglottis. The supraglottic larynx is the largest region and consists of the laryngeal surface of the epiglottis, the aryepiglottic folds, the arytenoids, the false vocal cords and the laryngeal ventricles.

The structures of the glottis include: the right and left true vocal cords, and the anterior and posterior commissures. The majority of glottic lesions arise from the anterior one-half of the vocal cords. The anterior commissure is usually within 1.0 cm from the skin surface. Because of this location, special attention must be given to the anterior border when designing the treatment portal for glottic cancers.

The subglottis extends from 0.5 cm below the glottis to the lower margin of the cricoid cartilage and is generally 1.5 cm in length.

Subdivisions of the Larynx (Left Lateral View)

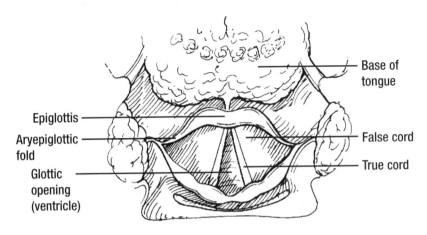

Base of tongue

Epiglottis

Aryepiglottic fold

Glottic opening (ventricle)

False cord

True cord

Fig. 1.13 The Larynx (Superior View)

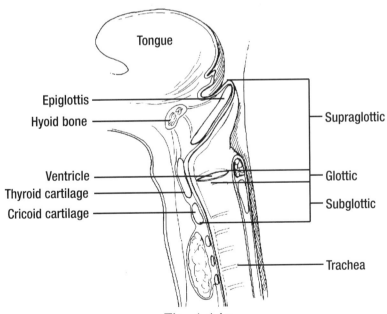

Tongue

Epiglottis

Hyoid bone

Ventricle

Thyroid cartilage

Cricoid cartilage

Supraglottic

Glottic

Subglottic

Trachea

Fig. 1.14a

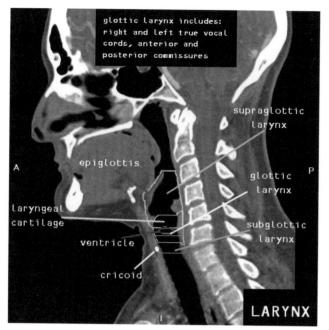

Fig. 1.14b

Routes of Spread

There are no capillary lymphatics in the true vocal cords.
Therefore, lymph node metastases do not occur until the
tumor spreads beyond the true vocal cords. The incidence
of lymph node metastases for a tumor confined to the true
vocal cords is 0-2%. For advanced disease the incidence
increases to 10-20%. Tumors of the supraglottic larynx
present with lymph node metastases 55% of the time, with
the first echelon of nodal drainage being the jugulodigastric
and the midjugular lymph nodes.

Glottic tumors often spread by local invasion to the
supraglottic or subglottic regions. Impairment in the
mobility of the vocal cords may occur by direct invasion of
the tumor into the underlying intrinsic muscle
(thyroarytenoid). Vocal cord immobility is a poor prognostic

indicator. The incidence of distant metastases is 10-20% with the lung being the most common site for metastatic disease.

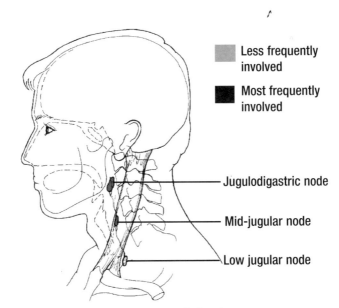

Fig. 1.15 Lymph Drainage of the Larynx

Treatment of Glottic Cancer

The goal of therapy for laryngeal cancer is curative treatment with minimal functional impairment. Treatment options for early glottic lesions include external beam radiation, hemi-laryngectomy, cordectomy or transoral removal of the lesion. Radiation therapy is the preferred treatment in early stage tumors to preserve voice quality with excellent cure rates. Surgery is generally reserved for salvage.

Technical Aspects of Radiation Therapy

For a T1 lesion (confined to the vocal cord), the portal is limited to the vocal cords. The lymphatics are not electively treated since the risk of involvement is only 0-2%.

The glottic larynx is treated through parallel opposed lateral fields. The borders, which can be clinically palpated, are described below:

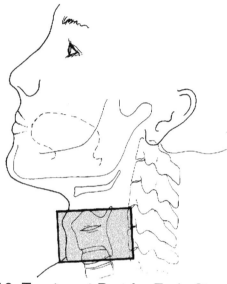

Fig. 1.16 Treatment Port for Early Stage Larynx

Anterior: 1.5-2 cm beyond the thyroid cartilage
Superior: top of thyroid cartilage
Posterior: anterior margin of the vertebral bodies
Inferior: below the cricoid cartilage

For T2 lesions, with normal cord mobility and minimal tumor extension, treatment portals are designed with a 2-3 cm margin around the tumor. Depending on the extent of the lesion, the jugulodigastric and midjugular nodes may be covered in the treatment port, especially in patients with impaired cord mobility.

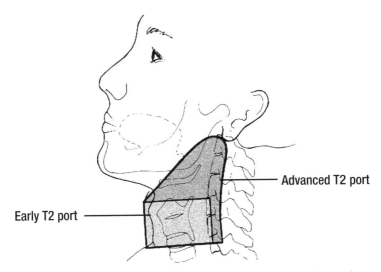

Fig. 1.17 Treatment Borders for T2 Tumors of the Larynx

Superior: supraglottic extension and 2-3 cm margin
Anterior: 1.5-2 cm beyond the thyroid cartilage
Posterior: mid-vertebral bodies
Inferior: infraglottic extension and 2-3 cm margin

Advanced or bulky lesions of the glottic larynx (T3 and T4: cord fixation, destruction of cartilage, or extension beyond the larynx) are best treated with total laryngectomy. Postoperative radiation is administered if indicated.

Patients on protocol are presently undergoing trials of chemotherapy and radiation versus radiation alone for patients with fixed vocal cords (T3). Radiation may also be used for palliation in inoperable patients.

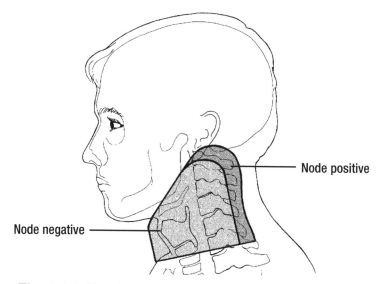

Fig. 1.18 Borders for T3/T4 or Node Positive Larynx

Anterior: 1.5-2 cm beyond the thyroid cartilage
Posterior: *node negative* - behind the mastoid process to
include the midjugular nodes
node positive - behind the spinous process to
include the posterior cervical lymph nodes
Superior: *node negative* - 2 cm above the angle of the
mandible to treat the jugulodigastric nodes
node positive - above the mastoid process to cover
the entire jugulodigastric lymph node chain.
(The hyoid bone and epiglottis are included to
incorporate the pre-epiglottic space)
Inferior: below the cricoid cartilage or to include the
supraclavicular area

The supraclavicular and lower jugular lymph nodes can be
included with IMRT treatment of the primary, or a separate
lower neck field can be abutted to the primary field.

Treatment of Supraglottic Larynx

Early supraglottic carcinomas are best managed by external beam radiation or supraglottic laryngectomy. For early tumors with minimal local extension and normal cord mobility, radiation is advocated.

Bulky, advanced lesions, that have fixed cords, or cartilage invasion can be managed with total laryngectomy and radical neck dissection. Postoperative radiation is delivered when indicated. Advanced disease may be treated with chemotherapy and radiation versus radiation alone on protocol. Radiation may also be used for palliation in inoperable patients.

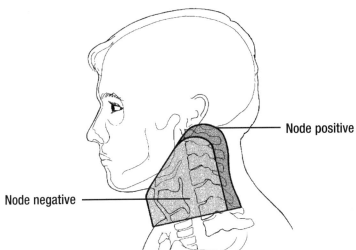

Fig. 1.19 Treatment Fields for Supraglottic Tumors

Anterior: 1.5-2 cm beyond the thyroid cartilage

Posterior: *node negative* - behind the mastoid process to include the midjugular nodes

node positive - behind the spinous process to include the posterior cervical lymph nodes

Superior: *node negative* - 2 cm above the angle of the mandible to treat the jugulodigastric nodes *node positive* - above the mastoid process to treat the entire jugulodigastric lymph node chain (the hyoid bone and epiglottis are included to incorporate the pre-epiglottic space)

Inferior: bottom of the cricoid cartilage and 2 cm below the lowest extent of disease

A boost volume should be designed to encompass the involved lymph nodes, and the primary tumor with a 1 cm margin.

Lower jugular and supraclavicular lymph nodes are treated for T2, T3 and T4 disease. The tracheal stoma should be electively treated in the anterior neck field in patients who have an emergency tracheotomy, or who exhibit subglottic extension, close or positive tracheal margin, or involvement of the soft tissues of the neck.

CT ANATOMY

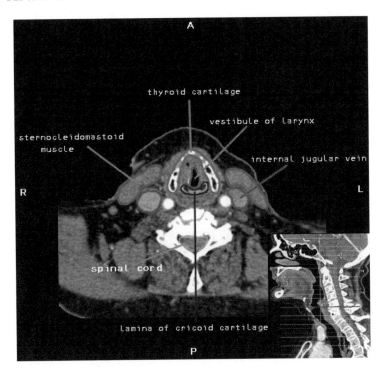

TOLERANCE DOSES

TD5/5 Normal Tissue Tolerances (Gy) 1.8-2.0 Gy/fraction				
Organ	1/3	2/3	3/3	End Point
Larynx (cartilage)	79	70	70	Cartilage necrosis
Larynx (vocal cords)	45	45	45	Edema
Spinal Cord	50 (5cm)	50 (10 cm)	47 (20 cm)	Myelitis/Necrosis
Thyroid	45	45	45	Thyroiditis

HYPOPHARYNX

The most common site for presentation of hypopharyngeal tumors is in the pyriform sinus, followed by the posterior pharyngeal wall. Postcricoid tumors are rare. 95% of hypopharyngeal tumors are squamous cell. These tumors are seen more frequently in men than women and are associated with alcohol and tobacco abuse. Patients often present with either a localized sore throat, a neck mass, dysphagia or ear pain.

Boundaries of the Hypopharynx

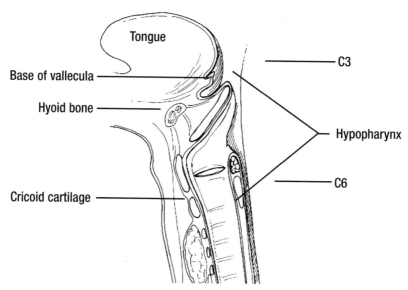

Fig. 1.20a

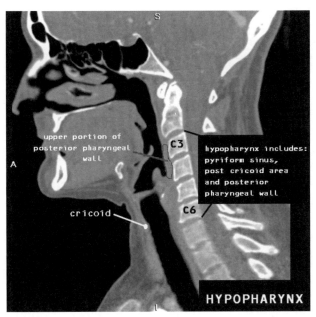

Fig. 1.20b

The hypopharynx includes the pyriform sinus, postcricoid area, and the posterior pharyngeal wall.

The superior border of the hypopharynx is the pharyngoepiglottic fold and the base of the vallecula which is located radiographically at the level of the hyoid bone.

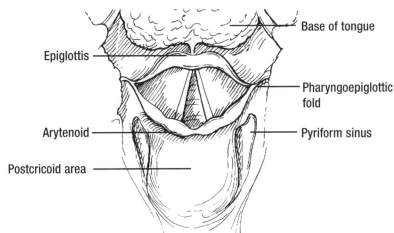

Fig. 1.20c Posterier View of Hypopharynx

The inferior border is the beginning of the esophagus which is at the lower border of the cricoid cartilage. The pyriform sinus has three walls and opens into the hypopharynx posteriorly.

Routes of Spread

The hypopharynx has a rich lymphatic supply. About 75% of pyriform sinus tumors, 60% of posterior pharyngeal wall tumors, and 40% of postcricoid tumors will present with lymph node metastases. The jugulodigastric and midjugular lymph nodes are most commonly involved as well as the parapharyngeal lymph nodes. Also, tumors may metastasize to the posterior cervical chain. At presentation, 20-30% of patients have distant metastases, with the lung being the most common site. Hypopharyngeal tumors also spread by local invasion.

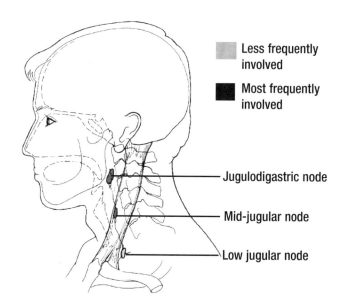

Fig. 1.21 Lymph Drainage of the Hypopharynx

Technical Aspects of Radiation Therapy

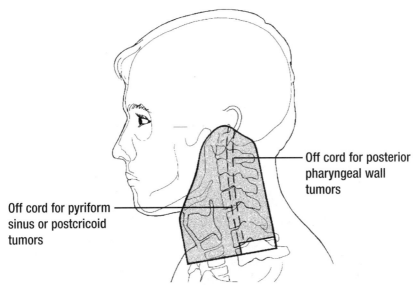

Off cord for posterior pharyngeal wall tumors

Off cord for pyriform sinus or postcricoid tumors

Fig. 1.22 Borders for Tumor of the Hypopharynx

Superior: inferior border of mandible and mastoid process (include margin on the jugulodigastric node which is located at the angle of the mandible), to the base of the skull (to cover the retropharyngeal nodes and the entire jugular chain lymph nodes).

Anterior: in front of the thyroid cartilage with a margin around tumor extension

Posterior: behind the spinous processes with a margin on all nodal disease (to include the posterior cervical lymph nodes)

Inferior: below the cricoid cartilage, to encompass the entire extent of the tumor with a 1.5-2 cm margin, or to include the lower jugular and supraclavicular area

The supraclavicular and lower jugular lymph nodes can be included with IMRT treatment of the primary, or a separate anterior lower neck field can be abutted to the primary field. If a separate anterior field is used, for postoperative treatment the spinal cord block should be placed in the lateral field so that the stoma may receive an adequate dose.

CT ANATOMY

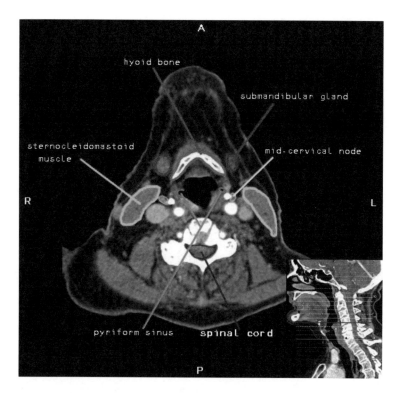

NASOPHARYNX

Although tumors of the nasopharynx are common in southern China, they are relatively rare in the United States. 85-90% of all nasopharyngeal tumors are epidermoid or undifferentiated carcinomas. Lymphomas comprise the remaining 10-15%.

Anatomy

The nasopharynx is a cuboidal structure with a rich lymphatic supply. It is bordered by the sphenoid sinus superiorly, the clivus and the first two cervical vertebrae posteriorly, the soft palate inferiorly, and the posterior choanae anteriorly.

An external landmark denoting the roof of the nasopharynx (or the floor of the sphenoid sinus) is the mid-zygoma which is a point midway between the external auditory canal and the lateral canthus.

Boundaries of the Nasopharynx

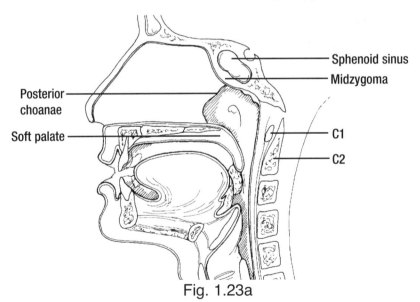

Fig. 1.23a

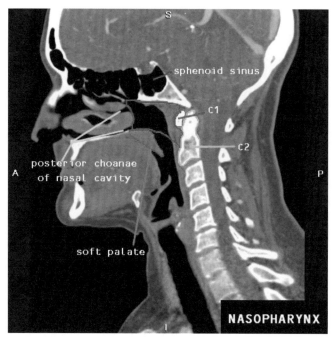

Fig. 1.23b

Routes of Spread

80-90% of nasopharyngeal cancers present with positive cervical nodes and approximately 50% of these will have bilateral nodal disease. There is no correlation between the size of the primary and the degree of lymph node involvement or the rate of distant metastasis. Nasopharyngeal tumors can also spread by direct extension. The sites for direct extension of the tumor include the tumor growing through the soft palate, into the nasal cavity, or through the base of the skull. Generally, the foramen lacerum is the opening through which nasopharyngeal tumors extend into the middle cranial fossa.

Lymphatic drainage of the nasopharynx is by three major routes:

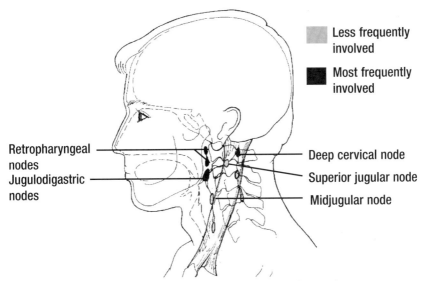

Fig. 1.24   Lymph Drainage of the Nasopharynx

1) the retropharyngeal nodes (retroparotid) - the upper most node in this group is the node of Rouviere. These nodes lie anterior to C1 and C2 vertebral bodies.
2) the deep cervical nodes (junctional nodes) which lie behind the sternocleidomastoid muscle at the junction of the spinal accessory nodes and jugular nodes.
3) the jugulodiagastric node

Technical Aspects of Radiation Therapy

Surgical resection of tumors of the nasopharynx is not possible; therefore, radiation therapy is recommended as definitive treatment.

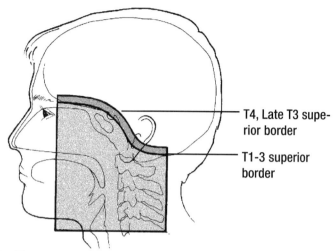

T4, Late T3 superior border

T1-3 superior border

Fig. 1.25 Treatment Volumes for Nasopharynx Tumors

The treatment volume for T1, T2, and T3 lesions (i.e., no base of skull or cranial nerve involvement) should include:

Anterior: posterior 2 cm of nasal cavity (or 2 cm beyond tumor extension). Posterior 1/3 of the maxillary sinus, posterior ethmoid sinuses, and the posterior 1/4 of the orbit

Superior: entire sphenoid sinus, cavernous sinus, base of skull (with at least a 0.5 cm margin)

Posterior: Behind spinous processes to include retropharyngeal nodes, posterior pharyngeal wall, deep cervical nodes, or posterior cervical nodes

In addition to the volume described above, the supraclavicular and lower cervical nodes should be treated because of the high probability of nodal spread.

For T4 tumors, the margins of the CTV should include the pituitary, and encompass all intracranial extension.

CT ANATOMY

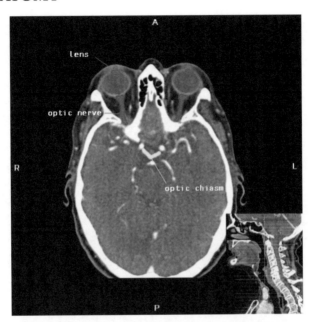

MR ANATOMY

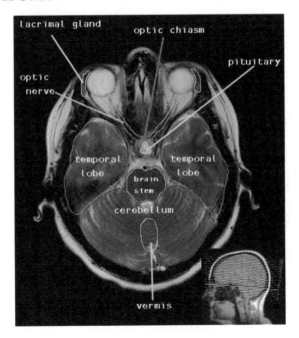

CT ANATOMY

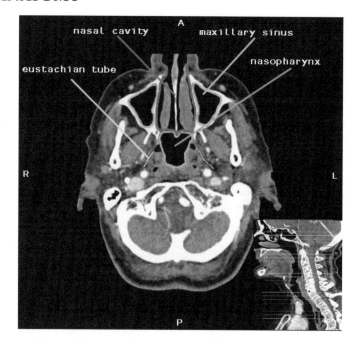

MR ANATOMY

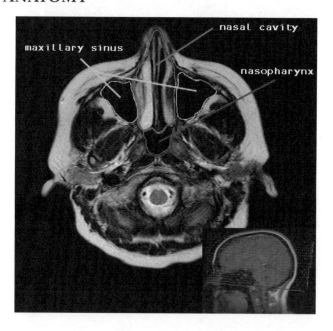

TOLERANCE DOSES

TD5/5 Normal Tissue Tolerances (Gy) 1.8–2.0 Gy/fraction				
Organ	1/3	2/3	3/3	End Point
Lens	10	10	10	Cataract
Lacrimal Gland	26	26	26	Dry eye
Optic Chiasm	50	50	50	Blindness
Optic Nerve	50	50	50	Blindness
Brain (temporal lobe)	58	51	47	Necrosis/Infarction
Brain Stem	60	53	50	Necrosis/Infarction
Spinal Cord	50 (5cm)	50 (10 cm)	47 (20 cm)	Myelitis/Necrosis
Parotid	32	32	32	Xerostomia
Ear	30	30	30	Acute serous otitis
Ear	55	55	55	Chronic serous otitis

NOTE: Qualitative Analysis of Normal Tissue Effects in the Clinic (QUANTEC) data suggests when sparing one parotid, the mean dose should not exceed 20 Gy. When both parotid glands are spared, the mean dose to both glands should not exceed 25 Gy.

L.B. Marks, et. al., Use of Normal Tissue Complication Probability in the Clinic, IJROBP, Vol 76, No. 3, Supplement 2010, S10-S19.

MAXILLARY SINUS

Of the paranasal sinuses, the maxillary sinus is most frequently involved with carcinoma. Histopathologically, 80% of maxillary sinus tumors are squamous cell, 15% are adenocarcinomas, and the remaining 5% are lymphomas, melanomas, or sarcomas. These tumors usually do not produce symptoms until they extend beyond the sinus walls.

Anatomy

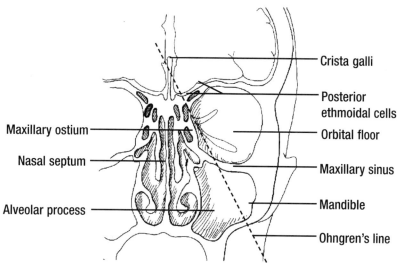

Fig. 1.26a   Anterior View of Maxillary Sinus

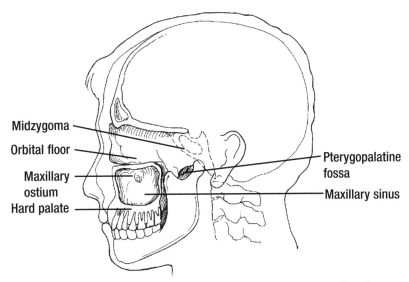

Fig. 1.26b   The Maxillary Sinus (Lateral View)

The maxillary sinus is bound by the following structures:

Superior wall: floor of orbit
Medial wall: thin walls of the nasal fossa
Inferior wall: alveolar process and hard palate
Posterior wall: posterior wall of the maxillary which separates the sinus from the pterygopalatine fossa and infratemporal fossa

Note that the floor of the maxillary sinus extends inferior to the floor of the nasal cavity and the roof is superior to the infraorbital rim. Also note the proximity of the posterior wall to the nasopharynx and the pterygopalatine fossa. These anatomic landmarks will be important for treatment set-up.

Routes of Spread

Tumors of the maxillary sinus are usually advanced at presentation with local invasion of bone. Tumors may present
with:

medial extension: through the nasal fossa, ethmoid or
                    frontal sinus (the maxillary ostium is a
                    pathway for medial extension) Patients
                    with gross disease in the
                    ethmoid sinusshould be considered to
                    have microscopic orbital extension
inferior extension: through the hard palate
posterior extension: into the pterygopalatine fossa or the
                    base of the skull
superior extension: through the floor of the orbit
anterior or lateral extension: through the walls of the
                    maxillary sinus to the cheek

Lymphatic spread from early carcinomas of the maxillary
sinus is rare. Once the tumor has extended beyond the bony
walls of the maxillary sinus the tumor is able to reach a
richer capillary and lymphatic supply. Overall, 8-15% of
maxillary sinus tumors present with lymphatic spread. The
pathways of lymphatic drainage depend on the area of
invasion. Lesions that invade the oral cavity and cheek
drain to the submandibular and upper jugular lymph
nodes. Tumors that invade through the nasal fossa and
nasopharynx drain to the retropharyngeal and superior
jugular lymph nodes.

Treatment

Initial surgical resection is recommended when possible.
Early infrastructure lesions may be treated with surgery
alone. Postoperative radiation therapy is generally recommended for all other patients. Patients who present with invasion through the posterior wall of the maxillary sinus (inva-

sion of the nasopharynx and / or base of the skull) are generally inoperable and must be treated with radiation alone.

Technical Aspects of Radiation Therapy

Treatment volumes are based on tumor extension. A tongue
blade is used to displace the tongue inferiorly from the
treatment field.

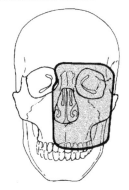
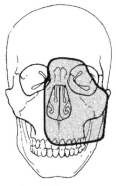
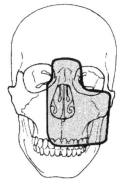

Fig. 1.27a	Fig. 1.27b	Fig. 1.27c
Orbital Involvement	Lacrimal Gland Block	No Orbital Involvement

Anterior borders:
The superior and lateral aspects of the field depend on the
extent of orbital involvement.

Superior: 2 cm above the cribiform plate (to cover the ethmoid sinuses)
no orbital involvement: include the floor of the
ipsilateral orbit but remain below the cornea
(Remember: the floor of the maxillary sinus
slopes upward). The patient should look straight
ahead to avoid overdosage to the retina.
orbital involvement: treat the entire orbit (with an
adequate margin around the tumor). Depending
on the extent of orbital involvement, the lacrimal
gland may be shielded at 40 Gy (unless the
shielding compromises the dose to the initial
gross tumor volume).

Inferior: lateral commissure of the lip (this will provide a margin on the lower border of the maxillary sinus) to include the alveolar ridge.

Medial: 1.5-2 cm across the midline to include the etmoid sinus and the medial aspect of the contralateral orbit

Lateral: to include the entire maxillary sinus tumor extent with an adequate margin (if the infratemporal fossa is involved, fall off is needed laterally)

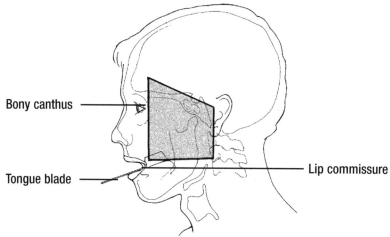

Bony canthus

Tongue blade

Lip commissure

Fig. 1.28   Lateral Borders of Maxillary Sinus Tumor

Lateral field borders:

Anterior: behind the contralateral bony canthus (the lateral portals can be angled 5 degrees posteriorly to shield the contralateral lens)

Superior: 2 cm above the cribiform plate and follow the floor of the cranium with a margin on the clivus

Posterior: include the pterygopalatine fossa and the nasopharynx with a margin on the posterior extent of the tumor. In patients with nasal cavity/nasopharynx involvement, include the retropharyngeal nodes.

Inferior: lateral commissure of the lip

Tissue tolerance of critical structures such as the contralateral optic nerve, and optic chiasm, lacrimal apparatus, spinal cord and retina necessitate tailored, planned dose constraints

Neck nodes are not routinely treated but should be included in patients with recurrent tumors, extension into the oral cavity, oropharynx, nasopharynx, or positive neck nodes. If the patient has had a lymph node dissection, the neck should be treated for multiple positive nodes or extracapsular extension. Bilateral lymph nodes are treated since the areas of invasion (oral cavity, oropharynx, and nasopharynx) are midline structures.

CT ANATOMY

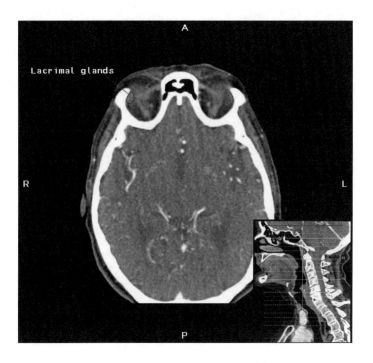

CT ANATOMY

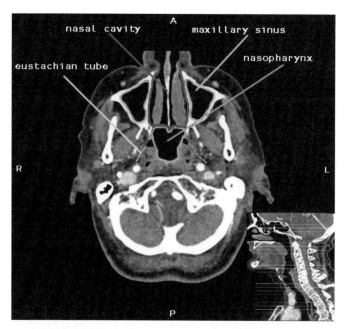

MR ANATOMY

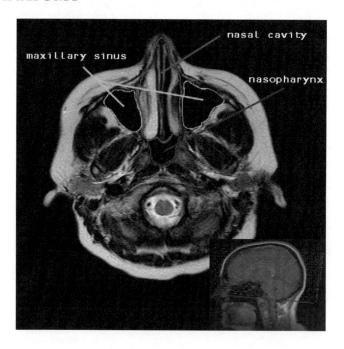

TOLERANCE DOSES

TD5/5 Normal Tissue Tolerances (Gy) 1.8-2.0 Gy/fraction				
Organ	**1/3**	**2/3**	**3/3**	**End Point**
Lens	10	10	10	Cataract
Lacrimal Gland	26	26	26	Dry eye
Parotid	32	32	32	Xerostomia
Spinal Cord	50 (5cm)	50 (10 cm)	47 (20 cm)	Myelitis/Necrosis
Temporomandibular joint	61	60	60	Marked limitation of the joint function

Note: Qualitative Analysis of Normal Tissue Effects in the Clinic (QUANTEC) data suggests when sparing one parotid the mean dose should not exceed 20 Gy. When both parotid glands are spared, the mean dose to both glands should not exceed 25 Gy.

L.B. Marks, et. al., Use of Normal Tissue Complication Probability in the Clinic, IJROBP, Vol 76, No. 3, Supplement 2010, S10-S19.

PAROTID

The parotid gland is the largest of the salivary glands. The majority of all salivary gland tumors, both benign and malignant, occur in this gland. The word parotid means "around the ear".

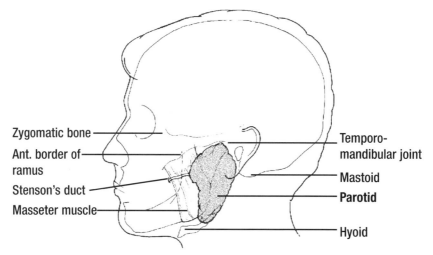

Fig. 1.29 Boundaries of the Parotid Gland

Anatomy

The parotid gland is shaped by the structures which sur-
round it. The superior border lies below the zygomatic arch,
and below and in front of the external auditory meatus. Posteriorly, it extends to the tip of the mastoid. Anteriorly, the
gland extends as far as the orifice of the parotid duct (Sten-
son's duct), which is adjacent to the second molar tooth. Inferiorly, the gland extends to the upper border of the posterior
belly of the digastric muscle, which radiographically lies
between the mandible and the hyoid bone. The facial nerve
artificially divides the parotid gland into superficial and
deep lobes. The parotid gland contains nodes within the sub-
stance of the gland and the first echelon of drainage is to the
ipsilateral jugulodiagastric lymph node.

Routes of Spread

The superficial lymph nodes of the parotid receive drainage
from the skin, subcutaneous tissue of the face, auricle, middle ear, and external auditory canal. Due to this drainage,

the parotid is commonly involved with metastatic disease as well as primary parotid tumors. Most malignant tumors spread through local invasion, ipsilateral neck lymph node spread, and perineural invasion. 25% of parotid tumors present with lymph node metastases and 25% have facial nerve palsy from the invasion of cranial nerve VII.

Technical Aspects of Radiation Therapy

The primary treatment for parotid tumors is surgery. Radiation therapy is indicated for: 1) high grade tumors, 2) positive margins, 3) perineural involvement, 4) positive neck nodes, or 5) recurrent disease.

The treatment volume includes the parotid bed and the ipsilateral upper neck nodes. For high grade lesions or positive nodes, the ipsilateral lower neck may be treated. If the tumor shows perineural invasion, the base of the skull should be included to cover the cranial nerve pathway.

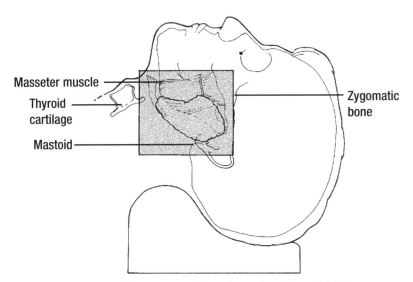

Fig. 1.30 Treatment Borders for Parotid Tumor

Superior border: zygomatic arch
(including all of surgical scar)
Anterior border: anterior border of masseter muscle
Posterior border: behind mastoid process
Inferior border: Top of thyroid cartilage

The parotid bed can be treated through an oblique paired wedge field, or by using mixed beams from a lateral field, or an IMRT technique.

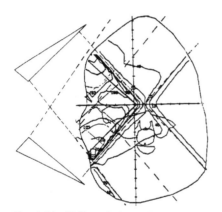

Fig. 1.31a Oblique Paired Wedge
Field for Parotid Tumor

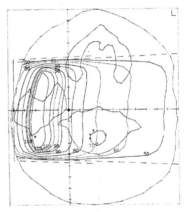

Fig. 1.31b Lateral Mixed
Beam Field

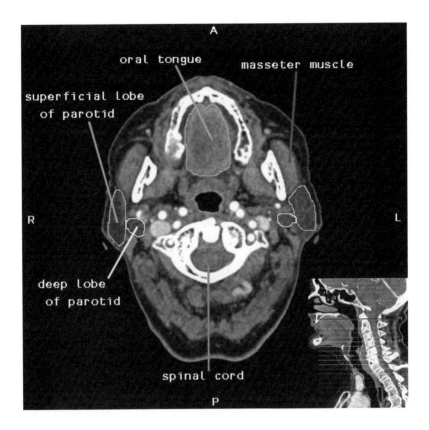

Head and Neck Treatment: Dose

A clinically negative neck (no evidence of nodal disease), which is at risk for subclinical disease is effectively managed with radiation alone. Doses of 50 Gy at 1.8 - 2.0 Gy per fraction are recommended. This is advantageous compared to a radical neck dissection because it offers coverage of all nodal areas treated and there is less disfigurement.

In neck nodes that are treated postoperatively, slightly higher doses may be needed, due to changes in the blood supply (less oxygen carrying blood for free radical formation). Clinically positive nodes measuring < 2 cm should be treated to 60 Gy, 2 - 3 cm nodes should be boosted to 70 Gy. In general, for nodes greater than 3 cm, preoperative or post-operative radiation is used.

Patients with borderline unresectable nodes should have lymph nodes boosted to 70 - 80 Gy, and resection should follow after radiation therapy.

Floor of mouth and oral tongue tumors can be treated post-operatively to 60 Gy for negative margins and 70 Gy for gross disease with lymph nodes treated according to risk of disease. Higher boost doses may be delivered with IMRT boost or implant if needed.

Dose planning with IMRT can be performed at standard fractionation, 1.8 - 2.0 Gy per fraction, with boost fields to higher risk disease.

A simultaneous integrated boost technique with IMRT can be used in appropriate cases. All high risk disease may be treated to 70 Gy at 2.0 Gy per fraction in 35 fractions, while intermediate risk disease is treated to 63 Gy at 1.8 Gy per fraction and low risk areas to 58.1 Gy at 1.66 Gy per fraction.

Chapter 2

Central Nervous System Tumors

HIGH GRADE GLIOMAS

Primary tumors of the brain represent less than 2% of all malignancies in the United States. Astrocytomas account for 50% of all primary central nervous system tumors. Astrocytomas can be divided into three categories: well-differentiated (mild hypercellularity and pleomorphism), anaplastic (increased pleomorphism and proliferative activity) and glioblastoma multiforme (tumor necrosis is present). High grade astrocytomas (anaplastic astrocytomas and glioblastoma multiforme) primarily occur in the elderly population, 50-80 year old. Overall the five year survival is less than 10%.

Anatomy

The central nervous system is composed of gray and white matter. Gray matter is made of oligodendroglia, astrocytes, and non-dividing neurons. White matter is composed of nerve fibers, axons, oligodendroglia, and supporting astrocytes. Astrocytomas predominately arise in the white matter. These tumors tend to present as a single mass arising in one hemisphere. Astrocytomas in adults most commonly arise in the cerebrum. 75% of astrocytomas are supratentorial. The cerebellum is the most common infratentorial site, and these tumors are more commonly seen in the younger age group.

Divisional Lobes of the Brain

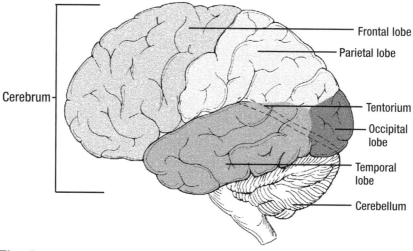

Fig. 2.1a

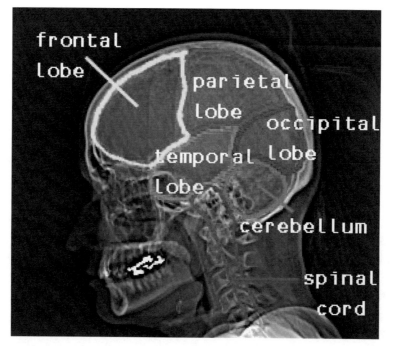

Fig. 2.1b

Routes of Spread

Gliomas primarily spread through local invasion along the pre-existing pathways defined by white matter tracts. The extent of infiltration may be a long distance from the primary tumor. Tumor cells have been found on biopsy series in the peritumoral edema. Anaplastic astrocytomas and glioblastoma multiforme may also seed the cerebrospinal fluid.

Treatment

For high grade astrocytomas, radiation therapy is delivered after biopsy or resection. Whole brain irradiation was advocated in the past due to both the infiltrative nature of these tumors and the fact that CT and MRI were not available for imaging. Since the development of CT and MRI, limited radiation fields encompassing the contrast enhanced lesion with a margin, have been advocated. Even though spinal seeding is a mode of spread, craniospinal irradiation is not advocated since local failure is the predominate problem. Limited field irradiation provides equal (although poor) survival rates compared to whole brain irradiation. With limited fields there is less damage to the central nervous system in the few long term survivors. Whole brain irradiation is reserved for multifocal lesions, or lesions with ependymal involvement.

Technical Aspects of Radiation Therapy

A 2-3 cm margin is generally placed around the contrast enhanced tumor volume and surrounding edema, using preoperative scans. Adequate coverage of the tumor volume may be accomplished with two or more treatment fields. Two or more fields in a 3D conformal, or IMRT plan, may offer sparing of the opposite cortex.

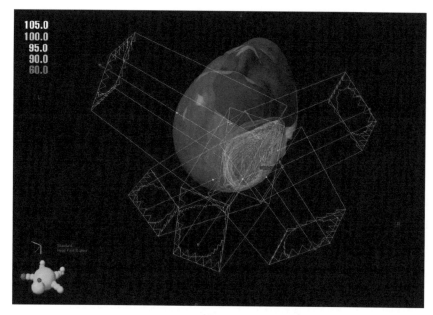

Fig. 2.2   IMRT for Glioma

Dose

Conventional radiation therapy doses for partial brain fields are standardly 60 Gy at 1.8-2.0 Gy per fraction. The portal may be reduced after 50 Gy, if the initial portal is large. The reduced portal should encompass the contrast enhanced tumor, not including edema, with a 2-3 cm margin.

PITUITARY TUMORS

About 10% of all symptomatic intracranial tumors arise in the pituitary gland. Asymptomatic adenomas are found 10-20% of the time at autopsy. Patients with pituitary adenomas may present with endocrine abnormalities as a result of hypersecretion of hormones caused by the tumor. Visual impairment, due to encroachment of the tumor on the optic chiasm, is another common presentation. Patients with large adenomas may also present with cranial nerve abnormalities due to encroachment on the cranial nerves which lie lateral to the sella turcica in the cavernous sinus.

There are three histological subtypes of pituitary tumors. The chromophobe adenomas, which are endocrine inactive, are the most common. Acidophillic adenomas may secrete growth hormone or prolactin. The third type, basophilic adenomas, may secrete ACTH, thyroid stimulating hormone or follicle stimulating hormone.

Anatomy

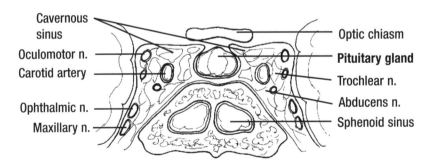

Fig. 2.3a Boundaries of the Pituitary Gland (Frontal Section)

The pituitary gland is a midline structure that lies in the sella turcica. The sella is a saddle-shaped cavity in the body of the sphenoid bone. Radiographically, the sella is located approximately 2 cm anterior to, and 2 cm above, the external acoustic meatuses. The sphenoid sinus lies below the pituitary. The cavernous sinus is lateral to the pituitary and contains the internal carotid artery and the cranial nerves III, IV, and VI which innervate the eye muscles. This sinus also contains the ophthalmic and maxillary branches of cranial nerve V which supply sensory to the skin of the face. The optic chiasm is usually located anterior and superior to the pituitary.

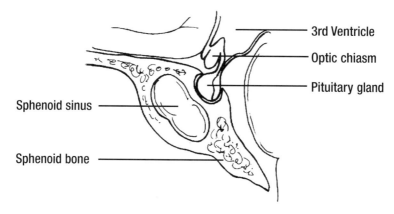

Fig. 2.3a Boundaries of the Pituitary Gland (Sagittal Section)

Routes of Spread

Pituitary adenomas are histologically benign and do not spread through the lymphatics or the bloodstream; however, they can cause damage by local invasion and compression. Tumors which invade laterally into the cavernous sinus may present with extraocular muscle dysfunction from compression of cranial nerves III, IV, and VI. Optic nerve compression may cause bilateral visual loss (bitemporal hemianopsia). Local invasion may also cause headaches, increased intracranial pressure, or cerebrospinal fluid rhinorrhea (from the downward extension of tumor through the sphenoid sinus).

Treatment

Pituitary adenomas are divided into micro- or macroadenomas. Microadenomas are less than 10 mm in size. Microadenomas may be treated with surgery through a transphe-
noidal resection. Larger tumors may require a craniotomy
for removal.

Radiation therapy may be used for definitive treatment or
postoperatively. In general, radiation therapy controls
hypersecretion in 80% of patients with increased growth
hormone, 50-80% with increased ACTH, and 33% with
increased secretion of prolactin. However, with radiation,
normalization of hormone levels may require months to one
year. Patients with a mass effect should undergo surgical
decompression to reverse symptoms.

Postoperative radiation is generally recommended after
subtotal resection of macroadenomas. It is also recommended after gross total removal of the tumor if there is persis-
tent hormone elevation (consistent with residual disease), or
recurrent tumors.

Technical Aspects of Radiation Therapy

Since the pituitary gland is a small midline tumor, the goal
of treatment is to deliver a homogeneous dose to the preoperative adenoma and spare normal brain tissue. This is best
done through multiple fields (two laterals and a vertex
field), or arcs.

The target volume for the field should be enclosed within
the 95% isodose line. For arc therapy, the patient is supine
with the chin tucked so that when the gantry rotates, the
beam does not traverse the superior orbit. This position can
be achieved by elevating the patient's head with a head

holder, or by placing the patient on a slant board. The field is generally centered on the sella, measuring 5x5 cm to 6x6 cm in size. A 3D conformal, or an IMRT plan, can be used to deliver a homogeneous dose distribution.

CT ANATOMY

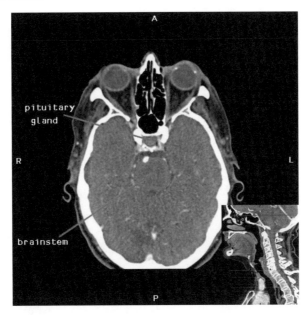

MR ANATOMY

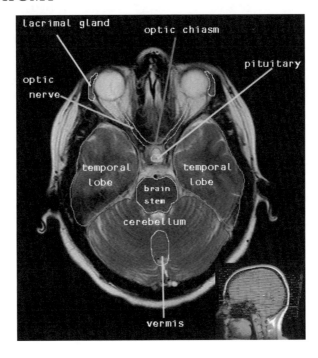

TOLERANCE DOSES

TD5/5 Normal Tissue Tolerances (Gy) 1.8–2.0 Gy/fraction				
Organ	1/3	2/3	3/3	End Point
Lens	10	10	10	Cataract
Lacrimal Gland	26	26	26	Dry eye
Optic Chiasm	50	50	50	Blindness
Optic Nerve	50	50	50	Blindness
Brain (temporal lobe)	58	51	47	Necrosis/Infarction
Brain Stem	60	53	50	Necrosis/Infarction
Spinal Cord	50 (5cm)	50 (10 cm)	47 (20 cm)	Myelitis/Necrosis
Ear	30	30	30	Acute serous otitis
Ear	55	55	55	Chronic serous otitis

Dose

The dose delivered is generally 45-50 Gy at 1.8-2.0 Gy per fraction, and larger masses may require a boost to 54 Gy.

Chapter 3

Breast Cancer

Breast cancer is the most common malignancy in women in the United States. One of every eight females will have cancer of the breast during their life. There is an increased risk of breast cancer in women with a family history of this cancer and in women who are nulliparous. Early stage breast cancer can be successfully treated with conservative surgery followed by radiation treatments. Conservative surgery followed by radiation provides the same curability as mastectomy but without the psychological and physical loss of the breast. Mastectomy should be reserved for patients with extensive carcinoma (unable to be resected with clear margins and an acceptable cosmetic outcome), or patients who prefer this alternative.

Breast cancer arises from the epithelium of the ducts. The most common histology is infiltrating ductal, which accounts for 65-80% of all invasive breast cancers.

Anatomy

The adult breast extends vertically from the second to the sixth costal cartilage and horizontally from the edge of the sternum to the anterior axillary line. Breast tissue extends into the axilla as the axillary tail of Spence. The deep surface of the breast lies on the pectoralis major and serratus muscles.

Routes of Spread

The breast contains lymphatics which drain through three major pathways: the axillary, the internal mammary, and the transpectoral. Breast cancer also spreads by direct extension or through the dermal lymphatics in all directions.

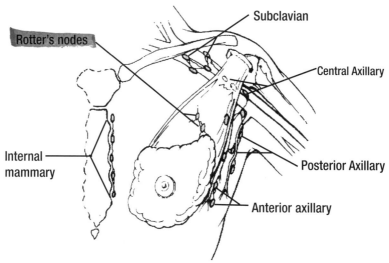

Figure 3.1 Lymph Nodes of the Breast

The internal mammary lymph nodes are located along the internal mammary arteries on both sides of the sternum approximately 3 cm lateral to the midline. They can be found at a depth of approximately 2.5-3 cm below the skin surface, in the intercostal spaces. The greatest concentration of internal mammary nodes is in the upper three interspaces. Involvement of the internal mammary nodes increases with central or medial tumors and proven axillary nodal metastases.

The transpectoral pathway passes through the pectoralis major muscle and drains into the supraclavicular lymph nodes. The supraclavicular lymph nodes are generally

located superior to the clavicle and lateral to the sternocleidomastoid muscle (at <3 cm below the surface).

The major route of nodal drainage is through the axillary
pathway. The axillary nodes are located near the patient's
midline, at a depth of approximately 6-8 cm. The axillary
lymph nodes are divided into three levels.

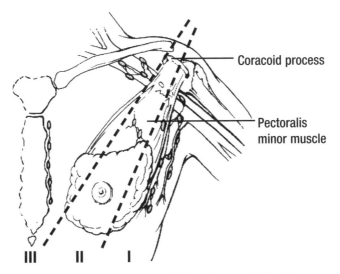

Fig. 3.2 Levels of the Axillary Lymph Nodes

Level I nodes under the lower portion and lateral to the
pectoralis minor muscle
Level II directly under the pectoralis minor muscle
Level III nodes superior to the pectoralis minor muscle

(Note: Level I-III nodes lie medial to the humeral head and
do not extend laterally beyond the coracoid process. The
nodes become more anterior as they extend superiomedial-
ly, i.e. levels I to II to III.)

Technical Aspects of Radiation Therapy

Conservative surgery and radiation therapy :

After wide resection with 1-2 cm margin of normal appearing breast tissue and an axillary dissection, the entire breast must be irradiated using tangential fields. A small margin of lung is included in the tangential fields so that the entire breast and chest wall are irradiated.

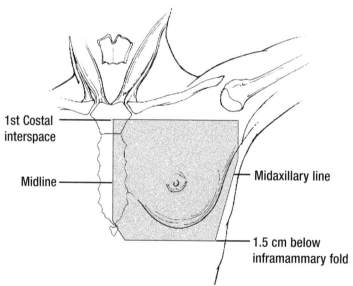

1st Costal interspace

Midline

Midaxillary line

1.5 cm below inframammary fold

Fig. 3.3 Tangential Irradiation Field

The breast tangential portals are set up with the following borders:

Medial: midline

Lateral: mid-axillary line (2 cm beyond all breast tissue)

Superior: first costal interspace (or as superior as possible, may be limited by the ipsilateral arm)

Inferior: 1.5 cm below inframammary fold

Generally, patients are placed on a slant board to compensate for the slope of the sternum and chest wall. In some cases, the slant board can also prevent the breast from falling superiorly toward the supraclavicular area.

A boost to the surgical bed is commonly recommended because microscopic tumor burden is greatest near the gross tumor mass. The boost may be given with electrons, reduced photon fields, or an interstitial implant. When using electrons the 80% isodose line should be on the chest wall, or below the deepest part of the tylectomy cavity. Be aware that the lumpectomy site does not always lie directly under the surgical incision.

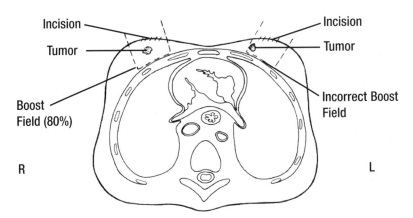

Figure 3.4   Comparison of Breast Boosts

CT ANATOMY

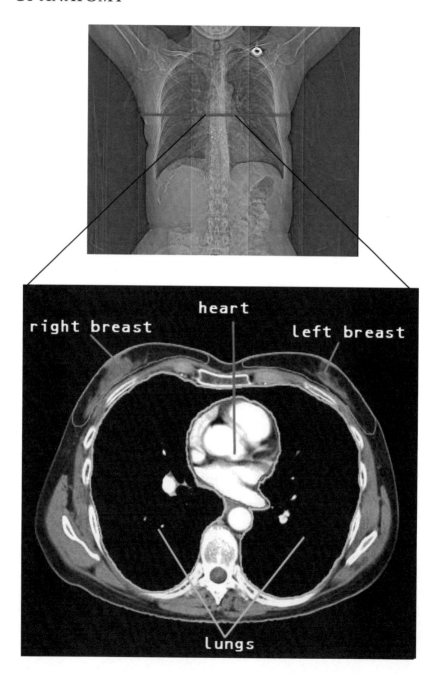

TOLERANCE DOSES

TD5/5 Normal Tissue Tolerances (Gy) 1.8-2.0 Gy/fraction				
Organ	1/3	2/3	3/3	End Point
Heart	60	45	40	Pericarditis
Lung	30-35	20-25	14-17.5	Pneumonitis
Brachial Plexus	60-62	60-61	55-60	Clinically apparent nerve damage

A supraclavicular field is generally treated in patients with four or more positive axillary nodes or extracapsular extension.

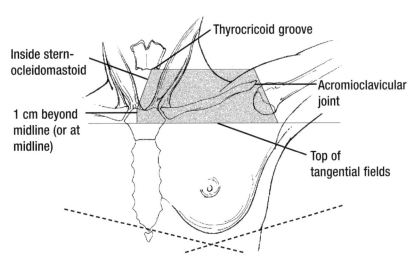

Fig. 3.5 Supraclavicular Irradiation Field

The supraclavicular field is set up with the following borders:

Medial: Vertical line 1 cm across the midline (or at mid-line) extending from the first costal interspace to the thyro- cricoid groove, medial to the stern-ocleidomastoid muscle to include the lower lymph nodes of the cervical chain. (These nodes lie under the sternocleidomastoid muscle and extend down to the insertion of the sternocleido-mastoid muscle at the head of the clavicle).

Superior: Extends laterally across the neck and trapezius to the acromial process (make sure entire supraclav-icular fossa is included visually).

Lateral: From the acromioclavicular joint, bisecting the humeral head, to exclude as much of the shoul-der as possible. A custom cut block may be used to block the entire humeral head. (Remember: the axillary nodes lie medial to the humeral head and the coracoid process).

Inferior: At the first costal interspace, abutting the tangen-tial breast field

The supraclavicular portal may be angled 10-15° to prevent exposure of the spinal cord and esophagus. The lower por-tion of the field is blocked with a matching half-beam block to eliminate overlap with the tangential field. When treating the tangential field, the table can be angled to match the superior border of the tangential field with the inferior bor-der of the supraclavicular field to further prevent overlap. Depending on nodal status, a posterior axillary boost (PAB), may be considered (see indications for a PAB in the Post-operative Radiation Therapy section).

Dose

The breast tangents should be treated to 46.8-50.4 Gy (at 1.8-2.0 Gy per fraction). Wedges, an intensity modulated segmented technique (i.e., field in field) or electronic tissue compensators can be used to achieve dose homogeneity and to reduce hot spots. Bolus is not recommended to the intact breast because the skin is not at risk for recurrence. The tumor bed is usually boosted to a dose of 60 Gy.

The supraclavicular field is generally treated with an anterior field to 46.8-50.4 Gy at 1.8 Gy per fraction.

Post-operative Radiation Therapy

Postoperative radiation adjuvant therapy after a modified radical mastectomy, is used to eradicate microscopic foci and increase local control in patients who are at an increased risk for local recurrence. The chest wall may be treated through tangential fields or single or multiple electron fields. If the surgical incision or drain sites extend outside of the treatment field, these areas can be treated with electrons. In general, the guidelines for chest wall irradiation are similar to treating the intact breast. For patients in whom the internal mammary nodes are not irradiated, the field borders are identical to Figure 3.5.

Treatment of the internal mammary nodes is controversial. Local recurrence in this area is low. Therefore, when treating only to prevent local recurrence, the internal mammary nodes do not need to be included. When treating a patient comprehensively and trying to affect survival, the internal mammary nodes are generally treated. The internal mammary nodes should not be included in the tangential fields on a routine basis because of the increased morbidity associated with including additional heart and lung in the treatment portal. Furthermore, by placing the medial border of the tangential field 3 cm across the midline in an effort to include the internal mammary nodes, there is an increased potential of irradiating the opposite breast, as well as an increased inhomogeneity of the beam. It is also uncertain whether the internal mammary nodes are adequately included when using this tangential method. In cases where the treatment of internal mammary nodes is indicated, a separate internal mammary node portal should be designed rather than exposing more heart and lung in the tangential field.

Various techniques have been used for irradiation of the internal mammary nodes concurrently with the chest wall. A commonly used method is described as follows:

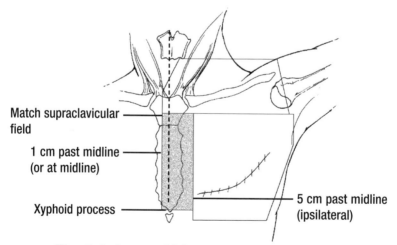

Fig. 3.6 Internal Mammary Irradiation Field

The borders of the internal mammary field are:
Superior: to match the supraclavicular field
Inferior: the xiphoid process

Medial: 1 cm past midline on the contralateral side
(or to midline)
Lateral: 5 cm past midline on the the ipsilateral side,
to include the internal mammary nodes

The tangential fields are matched to the lateral internal mammary port.

To prevent excess irradiation to the mediastinum, a mixed beam portal can be used to treat the internal mammary nodes. An electron energy should be selected to deliver 90% of the dose to 4 cm (usually 12-15 MeV). Remember: the internal mammary nodes are located at approximately 3 cm depth. The electron beam can be angled 5 degrees less than the medial tangential beam to decrease the cold spot between the internal mammary and tangential portals.

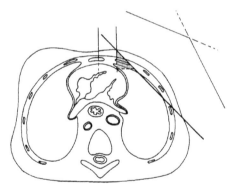

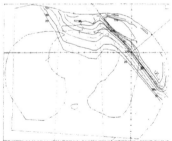

Fig. 3.7a Shaded area represents cold spot with anterior internal mammary node field.

Fig. 3.7b 5:1 15 MeV electrons: 6 MV photons. Electrons angled 5° less than medial tangential field. Note: No cold spot. Medial border is actually 2 cm contralateral to midline when angling the electron field.

The supraclavicular field should be set up as described in the conservative surgery and radiation therapy section. A posterior axillary portal can be used for patients with four or more positive axillary nodes, greater than 2.5 cm nodes, fixed nodes, extranodal extension, or an inadequately dissected axilla. This field is treated posteriorly to raise the dose in the midline and posterior axillary nodes that would have been underdosed because of the fall off of dose in the supraclavicular/axillary field.

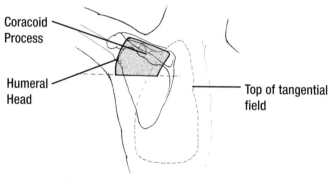

Fig. 3.8 Posterior Axillary Boost

The borders of the PAB are as follows:

Superior: bisect the clavicle and bisect the humeral head

Inferior: the field matches the superior border of the tangential field

Medial: to include the axillary nodes that lie close to the chest wall (a small margin of the lung is necessary). Remember: the level III nodes lie medial to the coracoid process and the level II nodes are medial to the humeral head

Lateral: the latissimus dorsi muscle

Dose

The chest wall is treated to 50.4 Gy (at 1.8-2.0 Gy per fraction). Patients with close margins, recurrent disease, or advanced primary tumors should be boosted with electrons to the surgical scar to 60 Gy. A 0.5-1 cm bolus may be used every other day (or every third day) to increase the surface dose to the skin. Use of bolus is especially important in patients with recurrent or inflammatory breast cancer.

The supraclavicular field is treated anteriorly to 46.8-50.4 Gy at 1.8 Gy per fraction. A posterior axillary field can be added to bring the deep axillary nodes to the prescribed dose.

Chapter 4

Hodgkin Lymphoma

Hodgkin lymphoma was first identified in 1832 by the pathologist, Thomas Hodgkin. There is a bimodal age specific incidence of Hodgkin lymphoma with one peak occurring between 15-30 years and the second after age 55. The World Health Organization (WHO)/ Revised European-American lymphoma (REAL) classification divides Hodgkin lymphoma into two main types: classical Hodgkin lymphoma (CHL) and lymphocyte predominate Hodgkin lymphoma (LPHL). The diagnosis of classical Hodgkin lymphoma is dependent upon the identification of the Reed-Sternberg cell which is a large, irregular cell with a multi-lobed nucleus. In LPHL, popcorn cells, or lymphocyte predominant cells are found without the Reed-Sternberg cells. LPHL is rare, and accounts for less than 10% of all cases.

The Ann Arbor staging system for Hodgkin lymphoma is based on the lymph node areas involved (I-IV) and the presence "B", or absence "A", of systemic symptoms which include fevers, night sweats and weight loss. Although the original staging system is still in use, there have been several modifications. Cotswold modifications to the Ann Arbor staging system incorporate factors which have been shown to effect clinical outcomes. These factors include introducing a category "X" to denote bulky disease greater than 10 cm, and identifying regions of lymph node involvement, denoted by an "E". Cotswold modifications added levels of response to treatment, and endorsed the use of CT scans to evaluate lymph nodes. The International Working Group (IWG) revised the Cotswold response to treatment category, omitting an "uncertain complete response" to therapy. PET scan results are now used to assist in the identification of residual disease.

The most common presenting symptom of patients diagnosed with Hodgkin lymphoma is a painless enlargement of a lymph node. Other symptoms which may be present and adversely affect the prognosis for early stage I and II disease are mediastinal adenopathy; B symptoms which include fever, night sweats and weight loss; numerous sites of disease; or significantly elevated erythrocyte sedimentation rate (ERS). Patients with stage III-IV disease are evaluated using the International Prognostic Score (IPS). This score helps to identify the treatment plan and the overall prognosis based on the number of adverse factors which are present at the time of diagnosis. The list of prognostic factors includes patient age, gender, stage, and specific blood values.

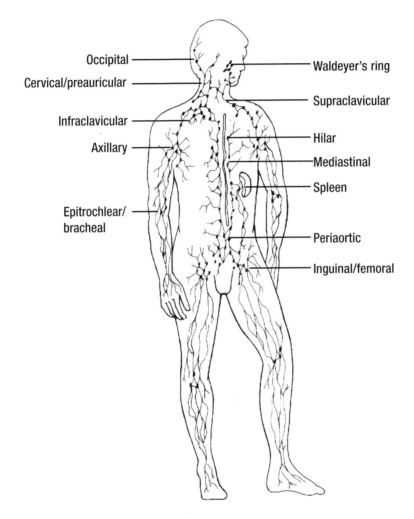

Fig. 4.1 Lymph Node Regions in Hodgkin Lymphoma

Treatment

The treatment strategy for Hodgkin lymphoma (HL) is influenced by the classification and subtype of HL, the location of the primary, the extent and stage of disease, and the patient's age and health status. At the time of diagnosis, classical Hodgkin lymphoma is usually found to be localized or involve contiguous nodal groups. At presentation, greater than 75% of the patients will have cervical or supraclavicular lymphadenopathy and 60% will have involvement of the mediastinum. The advent of the use of high energy x-rays, and of less toxic chemotherapy regimens, has resulted in a dramatic increase in the curability of this disease. It is now considered to be one of the most curable of all cancers.

Chemotherapy with involved field radiation therapy (IFRT), or chemotherapy alone, is often recommended for early stage classical Hodgkin lymphoma. Patients who cannot tolerate chemotherapy may be treated with extended field (regional) radiation therapy alone. Involved field radiation therapy covers only the lymph node regions with known disease, while extended field includes contiguous uninvolved lymph nodes. Chemotherapy is advocated for advanced stage Hodgkin lymphoma. It can be combined with radiation therapy for a large mediastinal mass, or bulky disease. Stem cell transplantation can be used for relapse or unmanageable disease.

Technical Aspects of Radiation Therapy (Extended Fields)

AP/PA Mantle Field

Treatment of the lymph node areas above the diaphragm is termed the mantle field. The nodal groups included in the mantle field are the cervical, submandibular, axillary, supraclavicular, infraclavicular, mediastinal, and hilar lymph nodes.

Patients are treated supine with their arms above their head, or on their hips, and their chin extended.

A typical AP and PA mantle port is shown below. In addition to the lung, humeral head and occipital blocks, anterior larynx and posterior spinal cord blocks are usually added. Modifications in portal size and field blocking can be made based on the stage and extent of the disease.

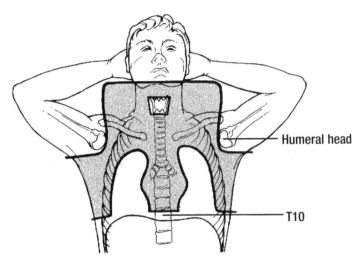

Fig. 4.2a Borders of the Anterior Mantle Port

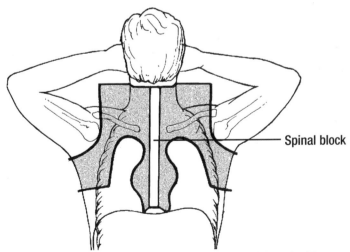

Fig. 4.2b Borders of the Posterior Mantle Port

Borders of the Mantle Field are:

Superior: lower mandible and the mastoid tips (the chin must be extended so that the high cervical and submandibular nodes are included in the port, without treating the mouth)

Inferior: T9-T10 interspace or insertion of the diaphragm

Lateral: fall-off, to include the axillary nodes

CT ANATOMY

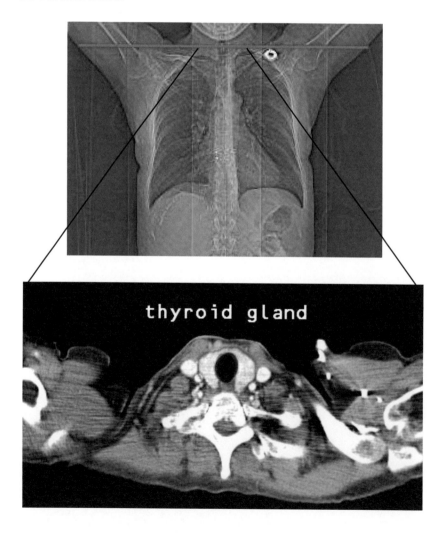

thyroid gland

CT ANATOMY

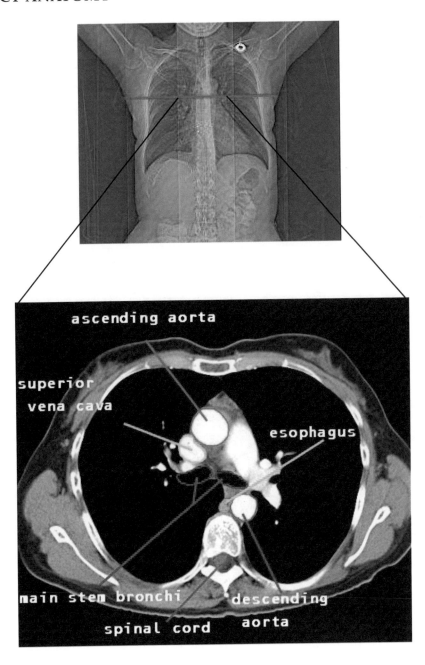

CT ANATOMY

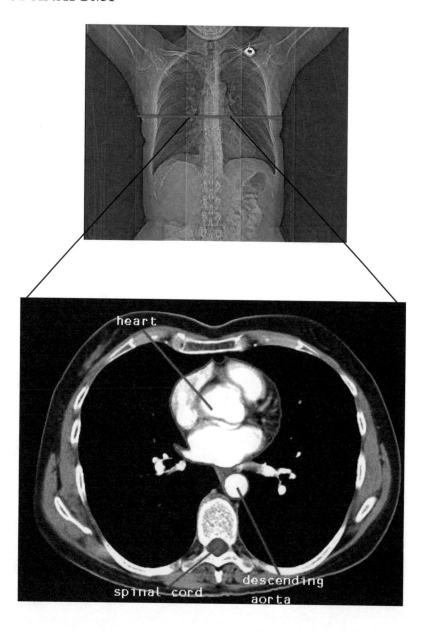

TOLERANCE DOSES

TD5/5 Normal Tissue Tolerances (Gy) 1.8-2.0 Gy/fraction				
Organ	1/3	2/3	3/3	End Point
Thyroid	45	45	45	Thyroiditis
Larynx (vocal cords)	45	45	45	Edema
Heart	60	45	40	Pericarditis
Lungs	45	30	17	Pneumonitis
Esophagus	60	58	55	Clinical stricture/ Perforation
Spinal Cord	50 (5cm)	50 (10 cm)	47 (20 cm)	Myelitis/Necrosis

AP/PA Inverted Y Ports

An inverted Y port consists of the following nodals groups: the retroperitoneal or periaortic nodes, the pelvic nodes, the spleen, or splenic hilar nodes, and the femoral nodes. When treatment of all of these areas is indicated, this large port is usually divided into abdominal and pelvic ports for sequential treatment. Separating the large treatment volume is usually better tolerated by the patient.

Subtotal nodal irradiation consists of irradiation of the mantle field and the abdominal (or periaortic) portion of the inverted Y. Addition of the pelvic ports to the mantle and the abdominal ports is termed total nodal irradiation.

If a mantle field was treated, the patient should be placed in the same treatment position. Precise calculation and verification of a gap must be recorded to eliminate any potential overlap of treatment fields on the spinal cord. In addition to the calculations and verification, a small spinal cord block may be placed superiorly at the junction of the mantle and subdiaphragmatic ports. Renal contrast is helpful in defining the lateral treatment borders, especially when the entire spleen must be treated. When treating the spleen, or splenic pedicle, the left kidney should be protected as much as possible. In certain cases, treatment of the liver is indicated.

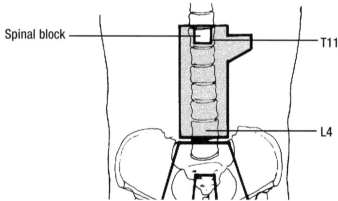

Fig. 4.3 Borders of the Abdominal (Periaortic) Port

Borders of the Abdominal (Periaortic) portion of the Inverted Y:

Superior: Approximately mid T-10, with an appropriate gap from the mantle field

Inferior: L4-L5

Lateral: usually 9-10 cm wide, (may encompass the spleen or splenic pedicle)

FEMALE PORT   MALE PORT

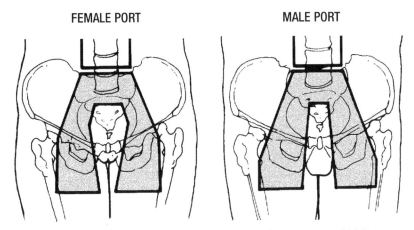

Fig. 4.4 Borders of the Pelvic Portion of the Inverted Y Port

Borders of the Pelvic Portion of the Inverted Y are:

Superior: L-5 with an appropriate gap from the abdominal port

Inferior: 2 cm below the ischial tuberosity to include the femoral nodes

Lateral: 2 cm beyond the pelvic inlet (exclude as much of the pelvis as possible while leaving an adequate margin around the lymphatics)

Treatment of the pelvis requires special consideration of fertility. Oophoropexy in the female as previously described moves the ovaries away from their normal position overlying the iliac nodes to a position in the midline which can be effectively blocked. In the male, blocking of the testes will reduce the integral dose.

Dose

Many studies and discussions have attempted to document the appropriate doses for Hodgkin lymphoma; however, controversy remains concerning the optimum total doses.

When chemotherapy is combined with radiation for
non-bulky, early stage I-II disease , doses of 20-30 Gy at
1.8-2.0 Gy per fraction are recommended. For all stages of
bulky disease (>10 cm in diameter) doses of 30-36 Gy are
recommended.

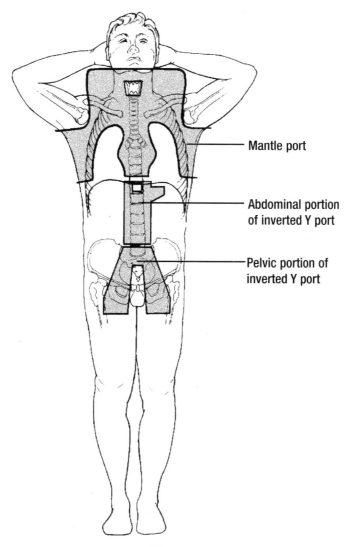

Mantle port

Abdominal portion
of inverted Y port

Pelvic portion of
inverted Y port

Fig. 4.5

Chapter 5

Lung Cancer

Lung cancer is the leading cause of cancer related deaths in both males and females. Approximately 16% of patients with lung cancer will survive five years.

Anatomy

The right lung is divided into three lobes and the left lung is divided into two lobes. The trachea branches into the right and left mainstem bronchi at the level of the fifth thoracic vertebra. The lungs are separated in the midline by the mediastinum which is composed of the heart, thymus, trachea, great vessels, esophagus, and lymph nodes. The mediastinum can be divided into superior and inferior compartments (above and below the level of the bifurcation of the trachea). The hila of the lungs contain blood vessels, bronchi and lymphatics.

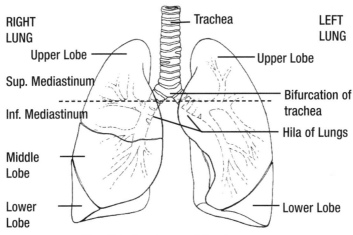

Fig. 5.1 Anatomy of the Lungs

Routes of Spread

The primary routes of tumor spread include the lymphatics, blood vessels and direct extension (intrathoracic). Involvement of the lymphatics tends to occur early and follows the divisions of the bronchial tree. The intrapulmonary nodes along the segmental bronchi are initially involved, followed by spread to the hilar nodes. The lymphatic channels then drain to the mediastinal nodes and ultimately to the supraclavicular nodes.

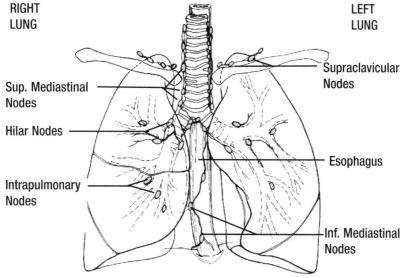

RIGHT LUNG

LEFT LUNG

Sup. Mediastinal Nodes

Supraclavicular Nodes

Hilar Nodes

Esophagus

Intrapulmonary Nodes

Inf. Mediastinal Nodes

Fig. 5.2 Lymph Node Drainage of the Lungs

Treatment Options

For general treatment purposes, cancer of the lung can be divided into two categories based on its histopathology: non-small cell and small cell carcinoma. In early stages of non-small cell cancer, when the tumor is localized, surgery is the treatment of choice. If the non-small cell tumor is inoperable (due to its size, location, or regional lymph node involvement) and has not metastisized, high dose radiation should be offered for optimal control. There is a direct correlation between the dose of radiation and local control in lung cancer.

Small cell cancer of the lung spreads rapidly, and has a high probability of metastasis at the time of diagnosis. Because of its rapid dissemination, multiagent chemotherapy and radiation therapy offer the best chance for a complete response. Many new protocols have shown a definite advantage to irradiating the chest simultaneously with the administration of multiagent chemotherapy.

Technical Aspects of Radiation Therapy

The treatment plan is designed based on stage, location, and lymphatic drainage of the primary tumor, and patient performance status.

Three dimensional conformal radiation therapy (3DCRT) has the potential to deliver high dose radiation (>70 Gy) to the primary tumor while sparing surrounding organs such as the spinal cord, heart, esophagus and normal lung tissue. A fourth dimension, motion management, employs techniques to account for tumor and organ motion during breathing. 4DCRT should be employed when feasible.

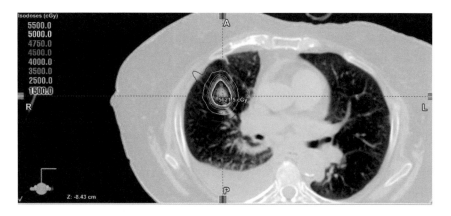

Fig. 5.3 SART for Lung Tumors

Stereotactic Ablative Radiation Therapy (SART), also known as Stereotactic Body Radiation Therapy (SBRT) is an image-guided approach using multiple beams to deliver higher doses per fraction, in fewer fractions, than traditional dose schemes. This technique is demonstrating improved local control rates in current studies.

For definitive radiation therapy with conventional fraction-ation, the inclusion of contiguous uninvolved lymph node regions is controversial. PET-CT scans are useful in identi-fying clinically involved lymph nodes to be included in the treatment volume, and concurrent chemotherapy allows for smaller radiation target volumes. The benefit of a reduced treatment volume is the ability to escalate the tumor dose while sparing normal surrounding tissue. The downside of a reduced treatment volume is a geographic miss due to motion and/or hidden disease.

CT ANATOMY

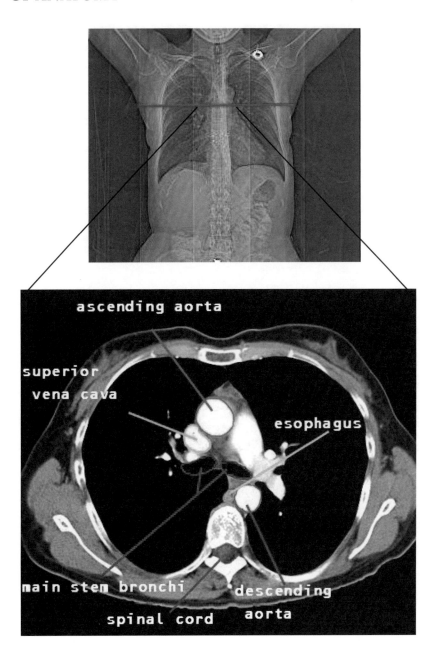

CT ANATOMY

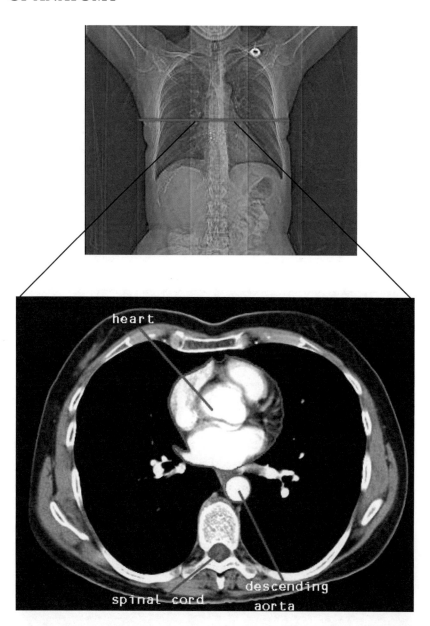

TOLERANCE DOSES

It is important to evaluate the dose volume histogram (DVH) to minimize normal tissue complications. The percentage of lung volume that receives xGy (Vx) is predictive in the risk of pneumonitis for the patient.

Prescribed Dose 30-35 fractions (1.8 – 2.0 Gy/fraction)				
Organ	**Suggested Tolerance**			**Endpoint**
Spinal Cord	Max ≤ 50 Gy			Myelitis/Necrosis
Lung	V5 ≤ 70%	V20 ≤ 30-35%	Mean ≤ 20Gy	Pneumonitis
Heart	V40 ≤ 80%	V45 ≤ 60%	V60 ≤ 30%	Mean ≤ 20 Gy	Pericarditis
Esophagus	Max ≤ 105% of prescribed dose	Mean≤ 34 Gy		Stricture/Preforation
Brachial Plexus	Max ≤ 66 Gy			Nerve Damage

Dose
Pre-operative doses typically range from 45-50 Gy in 1.8-2 Gy per fraction.

Definitive radiation therapy doses range from 60-70 Gy in 2 Gy per fraction.

Post-operative doses typically range from 50-54 Gy in 1.8-2.0 Gy to the tumor bed and high risk nodal area. A boost to 60-70 Gy may be delivered, but lung tolerance is lower and should be respected after surgery.

Chapter 6

Gastrointestinal Cancer

ESOPHAGUS

Cancer of the esophagus accounts for less than 2% of all cancers in the United States. The prognosis for cancer of the esophagus remains very poor with overall cure rates less than 20%. The incidence for esophageal cancer is higher in males than females. The major histologic type of esophageal cancer worldwide is squamous cell carcinoma; however, adenocarcinoma accounts for approximately 80% of all diagnosed cases in the United States.

Anatomy

The esophagus is a hollow tube of squamous epithelium, measuring 20-25 cm. A muscular wall surrounds the inner mucosa layer. The esophagus lacks an outer coating, or serosal layer.

The esophagus is usually divided into :
1) the cervical esophagus - extending from the cricoid cartilage to the thoracic inlet (level of T1)
2) upper thoracic - thoracic inlet to the bifurcation of the trachea
3) middle thoracic - proximal half of the esophagus between the bifurcation of the trachea and the gastroesophageal junction.
4) lower thoracic - distal half of the esophagus between the bifurcation of the trachea and the gastroesophageal junction.

Anatomical Landmarks and Divisions of the Esophagus

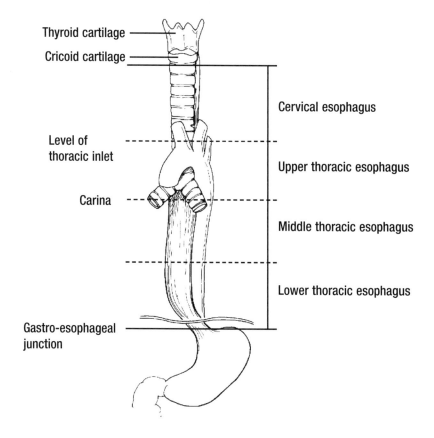

Fig. 6.1   Anatomical Divisions of the Esophagus

Routes of Spread

The esophagus contains a rich lymphatic network that interconnects throughout the length of the esophagus and generally spreads in a longitudinal course. Cancer cells may spread to any portion of the esophagus as well as to lymph nodes in the neck, thorax and upper abdomen. Tumors of the upper esophagus spread most commonly to the internal jugular, cervical, or supraclavicular lymph nodes. Middle esophageal tumors disseminate primarily to the supraclavicular, paratracheal and mediastinal nodes. Lower esophageal tumors generally involve the lower mediastinal, gastric, and celiac axis nodes.

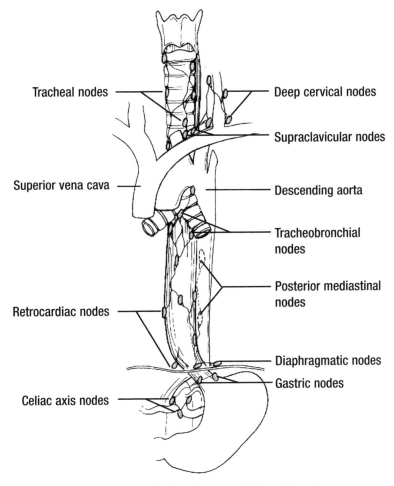

Fig. 6.2 Lymph Drainage of the Esophagus

Without a serosal layer, tumors of the esophagus may spread very easily to contiguous structures in the mediastinum. Also distant metastases via hematogenous spread is common and can occur early. Hematogenous spread to the liver, lungs and bones may be found in 40% of the patients at the time of diagnosis.

Technical Aspects of Radiation Therapy

Historically, if tumors were found localized in the esophagus with no evidence of metastases, surgery was the primary treatment. However, because of the high incidence of both local and distant spread, the results with surgery alone have been poor. External beam radiation therapy can be used alone in a curative manner for localized tumors or as a palliative measure to help relieve symptoms or obstruction. Recently, studies have combined chemotherapy and radiation therapy or chemotherapy, radiation therapy and surgery in an attempt to improve local control and cure rates. Patients who are found to have a complete response to chemotherapy and radiation have shown improved two and three year survival rates.

The primary tumor and involved lymph nodes (GTV) should be localized for radiation treatment. PET/CT scans, endoscopic reports, and diagnostic CT images are all useful studies. Areas at risk for microscopic disease should be identified and included in a wider margin (CTV) beyond the GTV. Due to the risk of longitudinal spread through a rich lymphatic network, an esophageal lesion generally includes at least a 5 cm cephalad and 5 cm caudal margin around the tumor and a 1.5 - 2 cm radial margin (PTV). Because of the close proximity of critical structures such as the heart, lungs, spinal cord, liver and kidneys, careful treatment planning and patient positioning must be observed.

Common treatment techniques include 3D conformal methods using multiple beam angles (e.g. AP-PA with oblique fields for a boost), or IMRT. When comparing 3D conformal to IMRT techniques, IMRT can often reduce the dose to critical structures while delivering the prescribed dose to the primary tumor and areas at risk.

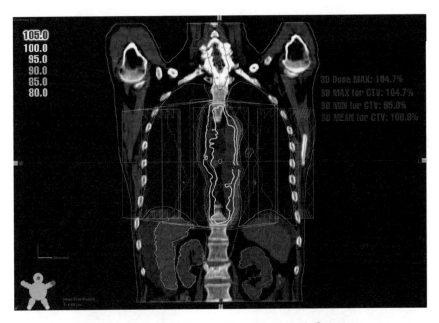

Figure 6.3 IMRT for Esophageal Cancer

CT ANATOMY

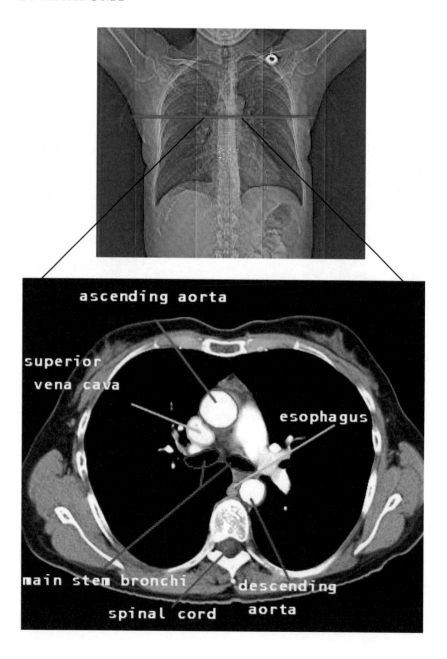

TOLERANCE DOSES

Suggested Tolerance Doses for Critical Structures near the Esophagus			
Organ	**Suggested Tolerance**		**Endpoint**
Spinal Cord	Max ≤45 Gy		Myelitis/Necrosis
Lung	V10 ≤40% V15 ≤30% V20 ≤20%		Pneumonitis
Heart	Less than 50 Gy to 30% of the heart (minimal dose to the left ventricle)		Pericarditis
Kidneys	Less than 20 Gy to at least 60% of one kidney		Renal insufficiency
Liver	Max < 30 Gy to 60% of the liver		Clinical hepatitis

Doses

45-50.4 Gy delivered in 1.8 – 2.0 Gy per fraction is recommended.

STOMACH

Although the incidence of stomach cancer is high in China, the incidence and mortality in the United States has declined over the past 50 years. Dietary factors such as smoked foods have been implicated as a risk factor in gastric cancer. Pathologically, most gastric cancers are ulcerative adenocarcinomas. Patients diagnosed with gastric cancer generally complain of weight loss, decreased appetite, abdominal pain and nausea and vomiting.

Anatomy

The stomach is made up of a muscular wall with a mucosal lining which contains a variety of different types of cells exhibiting different radiosensitivity. The stomach begins at the gastroesophageal junction and ends at the pylorus, which joins the duodenum. The stomach is surrounded by a number of vital structures including the liver, transverse colon, left kidney, pancreas, left adrenal, spleen, and segments of the small bowel.

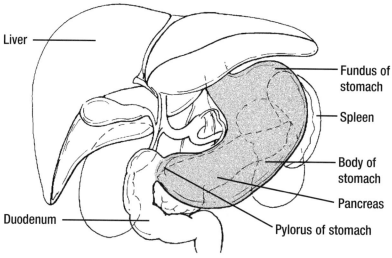

Fig. 6.4 Anatomy of the Stomach

Routes of Spread

There are four primary routes of spread for gastric carcinoma. These tumors can spread by direct extension to adjacent organs and viscera. Widespread dissemination occurs by way of the lymphatics, hematogenous spread, or by spillage into the peritoneal cavity.

The stomach contains a rich lymphatic network that connects and flows through three major pathways. The lymphatics can drain through the left gastric trunk, the splenic collecting trunk, or the hepatic collecting trunk. Splenic nodal groups that are at risk for metastatic spread include the gastric, gastropancreatic, celiac axis, and the adjacent periaortic nodes.

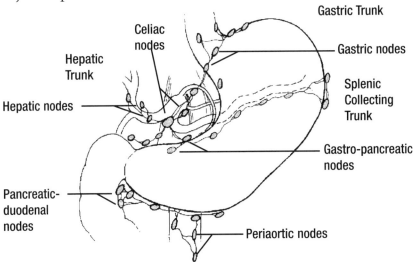

Fig. 6.5 Lymph Drainage of the Stomach

Treatment

In cases where the tumor is limited to the stomach, the treatment of choice is a radical subtotal gastrectomy with the removal of adjacent nodal tissue. Gastric cancer has a high propensity for locoregional failure. The tumor bed and regional lymph nodes are at greatest risk for recurrence. Distant metastases are also common with advanced disease, and often involve the liver and lungs.

Because of the high rate of locoregional failure following surgery, especially in cases where the tumor extends through the wall of the stomach or positive lymph nodes are found, radiation therapy has been used postoperatively. Post-op radiation, usually combined with chemotherapy, has proven to be beneficial in local control of the primary tumor. In unresectable cases, radiation has been successful in the palliation of gastric cancer symptoms.

Technical Aspects of Radiation Therapy

Radiation portals must be designed with careful consideration of the surrounding dose limiting structures. The radiation portal should include the tumor bed and the major surrounding lymphatic groups. Multi-field 3D conformal techniques to include AP/PA, four fields using AP/PA and opposed lateral beams, or an IMRT technique can be used.

Treatment Borders for Cancer of the Stomach:

Superior: 3-4 cm margin around the tumor or tumor bed
Inferior: bottom of L3
Lateral: 3-4 cm margin around the tumor or tumor bed and primary nodal groups with special contouring of the port to exclude three-fourths of one kidney

It is important to consider respiratory motion and stomach filling (if the stomach is intact) when determining treatment margins

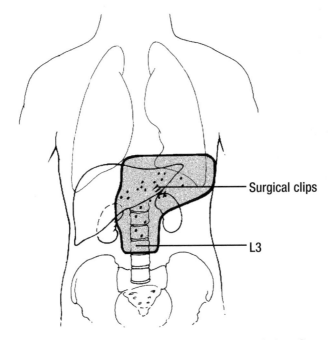

Fig 6.6 Postoperative Portal for Cancer of the Stomach

CT and MR ANATOMY *(diagrams on next page)*

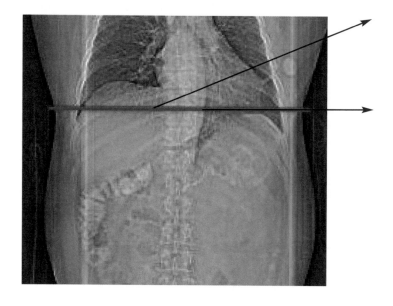

CT ANATOMY

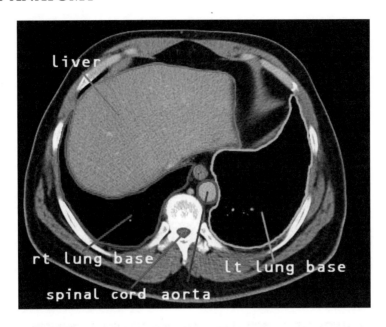

MR ANATOMY

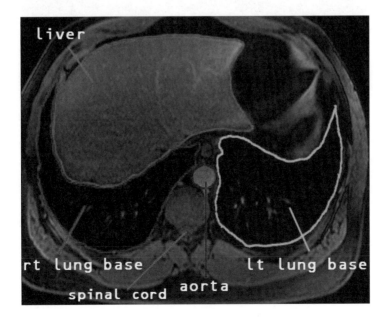

CT and MR ANATOMY *(MR diagram continued on next page)*

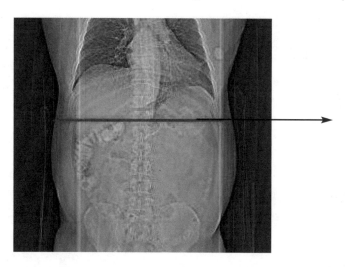

CT ANATOMY

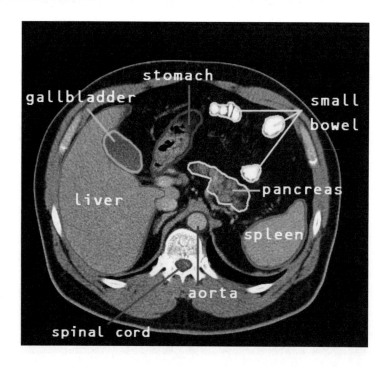

MR ANATOMY

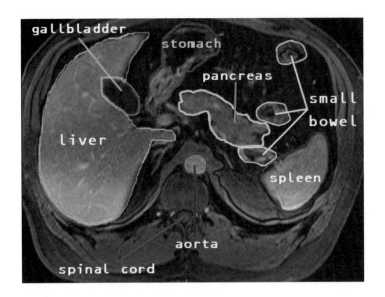

TOLERANCE DOSES

Suggested Tolerance Doses for Critical Structures near the Stomach			
Organ	**Suggested Tolerance**		**Endpoint**
Spinal Cord	Max ≤45 Gy		Myelitis/Necrosis
Lung	V10 ≤40%	V15 ≤30%	V20 ≤20%	Pneumonitis
Heart	Less than 50 Gy to 30% of the heart (minimal dose to the left ventricle)		Pericarditis
Kidneys	Less than 20 Gy to at least 60% of one kidney		Renal insufficiency
Liver	Max <30 Gy to 60% of the liver		Clinical hepatitis

Dose

45-50.4 Gy at 1.8 Gy per day is recommended.

PANCREAS

The incidence and the mortality rate of pancreatic cancer continues to increase and parallel one another very closely. Several factors associated with an increased risk of pancreatic cancer include cigarette smoking, alcohol consumption, and chronic pancreatitis. The majority of pancreatic cancers are ductal adenocarcinomas and occur in the head of the pancreas.

Anatomy

The pancreas is found in the posterior peritoneum. It is composed of three parts designated the head, the body and the tail. The head of the pancreas is overlapped by the duodenum at approximately the level of the first two lumbar vertebrae. The tail of the pancreas extends to the splenic hilum.

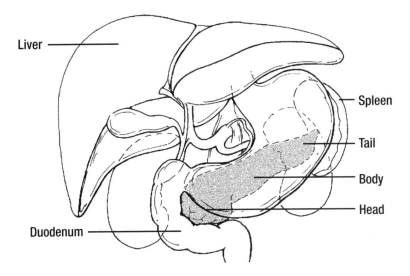

Fig. 6.7   The Pancreas

Routes of Spread

Because of the rich lymphatic network of the pancreas, several nodal groups are at risk for metastatic involvement. Those at greatest risk include the superior and inferior pancreaticoduodenal, the porta hepatis, the suprapancreatic and the adjacent periaortic nodes. Pancreatic tumors tend to spread by direct extension to adjacent vital structures including the bile duct system, the stomach and the duodenum. Hematogenous metastases are common and usually involve the liver, lungs or pleura.

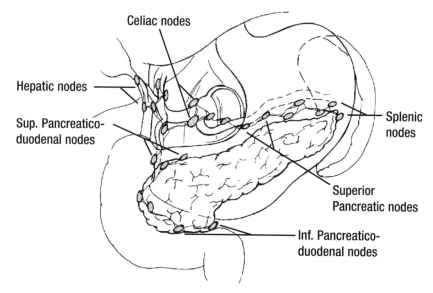

Fig. 6.8 Lymph Drainage of the Pancreas

Treatment

The treatment of choice for localized pancreatic cancer is surgical resection. Unfortunately, only about 10-25% of patients are candidates for surgery with curative intent. To date, 5 year survival rates remain very poor (5-10%).

For patients able to undergo surgery, there is evidence to support the use of postoperative radiation therapy in combination with chemotherapy. By irradiating the tumor bed and surrounding nodal areas, the risk of local recurrence can be decreased and survival possibly improved.

For patients with unresectable pancreatic cancers, palliation can be achieved using combined external beam radiation and chemotherapy.

Technical Aspects of Radiation Therapy

Due to the proximity of the pancreas to critical dose limiting structures (such as the liver, small bowel, stomach, kidney and spinal cord), multiple fields to include 3D conformal, IMRT, or volumetric modulated arc therapy should be employed.

The treatment volume can be determined by post-surgical clips, MRI or CT scans with the patient in the treatment position, endoscopic studies, or ultrasonography. The patient should be treated supine. A 2-3 cm margin should be planned around the tumor bed, or primary tumor, to include adjacent pancreatic tissue and major nodal groups. Renal contrast is necessary for precise localization of the kidneys, and barium can be used to delineate the duodenum. The portal should be planned to respect the tolerance of all surrounding radiosensitive structures, particularly the liver, kidneys and small bowel.

Treatment Borders for Tumors Involving the Head of the Pancreas:

The treatment portal for tumors located in the head of the pancreas should include the following nodal groups: the pancreaticoduodenal, the porta hepatis, the celiac, and the suprapancreatic.

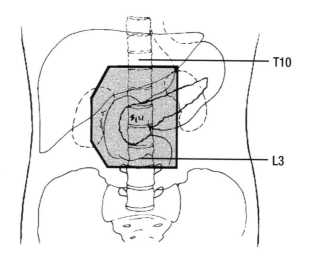

Fig. 6.9a AP Treatment Port for Tumor in Head of Pancreas

Borders for the AP or AP/PA port(s):

Superior: T11-T12 or a 2-3 cm margin around the tumor or the tumor bed

Inferior: bottom of L3

Lateral: 2-3 cm margin around the tumor or the tumor bed with exclusion of at least three-fourths of the left kidney. You may need to include at least 50% of the right kidney as well as the duodenum.

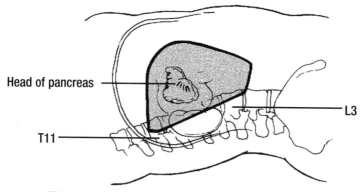

Fig. 6.9b Lateral Pancreatic Treatment Port

Borders for the Lateral Ports:

Anterior: 1-2 cm beyond the tumor or tumor bed
Posterior: split the vertebral bodies

Treatment Borders for Pancreatic Body or Tail Tumors

Treatment portals for tumors arising in the body or the tail of the pancreas should include the pancreaticoduodenal nodes, the porta hepatis nodes, and the splenic hilar nodes.

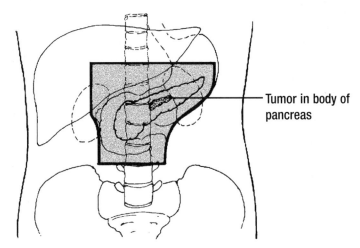

Tumor in body of pancreas

Fig. 6.10 Treatment Port for Tumor in Body/Tail of Pancreas

Borders for the AP or AP/PA port(s):

Superior: top of T11
Inferior: bottom of L3
Lateral: exclude at least two-thirds of the right kidney. It is not necessary to include the entire duodenal loop. The port is extended to the left to obtain a 3 cm margin around the tumor and to include the splenic hilum.

CT and MR ANATOMY *(diagrams on next page)*

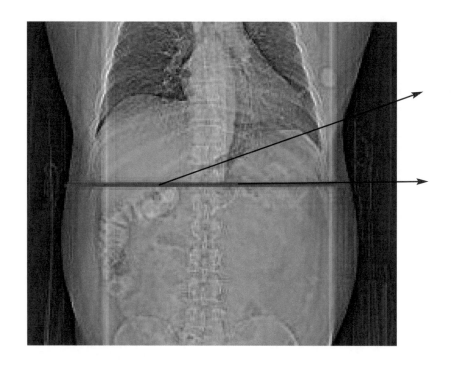

CT ANATOMY

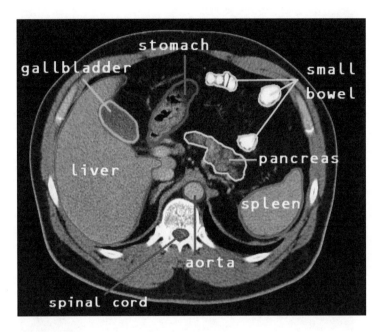

MR ANATOMY

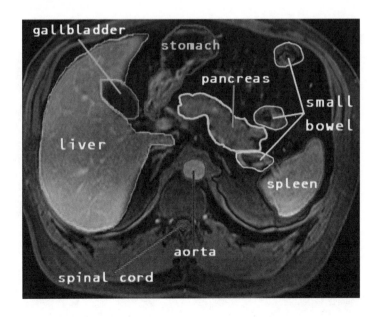

CT and MR ANATOMY *(MR diagram on next page)*

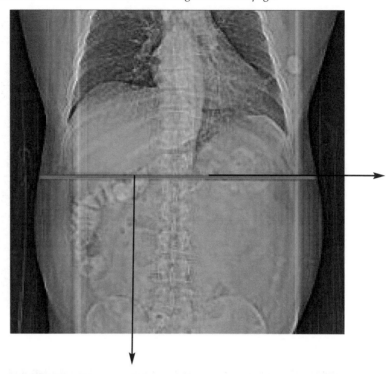

CT ANATOMY

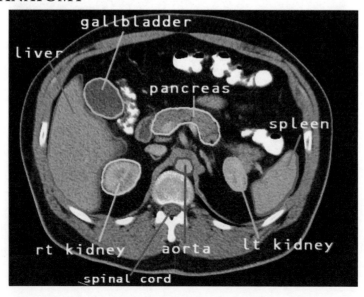

MR ANATOMY

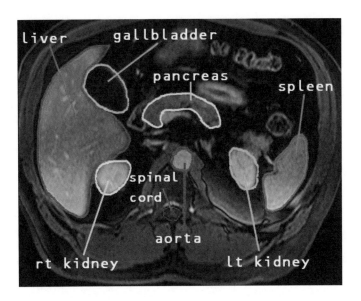

TOLERANCE DOSES

Suggested Tolerance Doses for Critical Structures near the Pancreas		
Organ	**Suggested Tolerance**	**Endpoint**
Spinal Cord	Max ≤45 Gy	Myelitis/Necrosis
Both Kidneys	Mean dose to bilateral kidneys should be 18 Gy. If patient has only one kidney, not more than 15% should receive ≥ 18 Gy and no more than 30% ≥ 14 Gy	Renal insufficiency
Liver	Mean dose ≤25 Gy	Clinical hepatitis
Stomach, duodenum, jejunum	Max dose ≤ 55 Gy; Less than 10% of each organ can receive 50-53.99 Gy. Less than 15% of each organ volume can receive 45-49.99 Gy	Perforation, stricture

Dose

For resected cases, 45 Gy is recommended to the tumor bed, surgical anastomosis and regional lymph nodes. A boost to 50-65 Gy may be delivered to the tumor bed and anastomosis, if critical structure tolerance is not exceeded. For unresectable disease, 50-54 Gy in 1.8-2.0 Gy per fraction is recommended.

RECTUM

In the United States, carcinoma of the rectum is the second most common cause of cancer related death. It occurs equally in men and women. The rectal cancer risk in women is slightly lower than the risk in men. The majority of rectal cancers are adenocarcinomas which arise from the rectal mucosa.

Anatomy

The rectum is located between the sigmoid colon proximally and the anus distally. It is 13-15 cm in length. The rectum can be divided into three sections by the upper, middle and lower valves of Houston. The rectum and sigmoid colon join at approximately the level of S3. The rectum is closely associated with the sacral curve posteriorly. It is bounded by the vagina anteriorly in the female and by the trigone of the bladder, seminal vesicles, and prostate in the male. The rectum ends distally at the pectinate or dentate line, where the transition from rectal mucosa to squamous epithelium occurs.

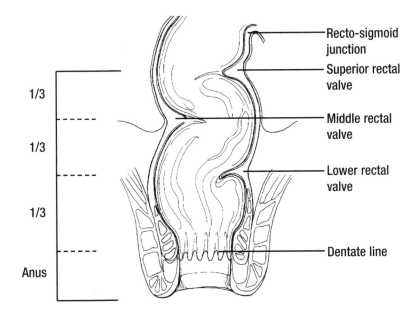

1/3

1/3

1/3

Anus

Recto-sigmoid junction

Superior rectal valve

Middle rectal valve

Lower rectal valve

Dentate line

Fig. 6.11   Anatomy of the Rectum

Routes of Spread

Rectal cancer can spread by four pathways. Spread can occur by direct extension through the bowel wall to contiguous structures or organs. Widespread dissemination occurs by way of the lymphatics, hematogenous spread, or by transperitoneal implantation at the time of surgery.

Longitudinal tumor growth within the bowel wall generally occurs only for very short distances. Rectal tumors most often grow in an angular pattern, with extension into and through the layers of the bowel wall. Lymphatic drainage for the upper rectum follows the superior rectal vessels and terminates in the inferior mesenteric nodes. The middle and lower rectal lymphatics drain to the internal iliac and presacral nodes. If the lesion extends to the anal canal the inguinal nodes may also be at risk. Hematogenous spread to the liver and lungs occurs most often with high grade tumors, and in those cases with lymphatic involvement. The liver is the most common site of metastatic spread.

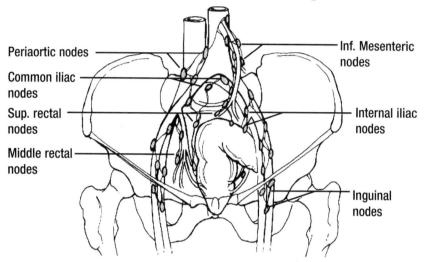

Fig. 6.12a   Lymph Drainage of the Rectum

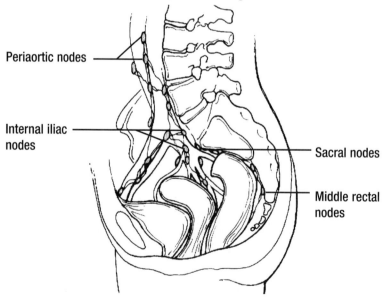

Fig. 6.12b Lymph Drainage of the Rectum (Lateral View)

Treatment

The treatment of choice for rectal cancer is surgical removal of the primary tumor and the primary nodal drainage. For tumors less than 6 cm from the anal verge, abdominoperineal resection with colostomy is required. In cases with rectal tumors greater than 6 cm from the anal verge, it is usually technically possible to perform a low anterior resection of the bowel with anastomosis. Local-regional failure is common in rectal cancer, especially for tumors extending through the bowel wall or involving regional lymphatics. For these reasons, radiation therapy and chemotherapy have been accepted as adjuvant treatment to improve the local control and survival of patients.

Radiation therapy has been used preoperatively, postoperatively, and both pre- and postoperatively (sandwich technique) in the treatment of rectal cancer.

Preoperative radiation therapy has the advantages of decreasing the viability of tumor cells that could spread at the time of surgery, improving the ability to resect large tumors, and decreasing the small bowel complications by radiating in a nonsurgical area.

Postoperative radiation has the advantage of better selection of patients for treatment based on the surgical pathologic findings.

Technical Aspects of Radiation Therapy

Whether preoperative or postoperative radiation therapy is used, the goal of treatment is to include the primary tumor or tumor bed with a 4-5 cm margin as well as the primary nodal drainage which generally includes the internal iliac and presacral nodes. The external iliac nodes are not generally included in the treatment port unless there is tumor involvement of other pelvic organs such as the vagina, bladder or uterus which may place these nodes at risk for metastases. In cases where postoperative radiation therapy is used following abdominoperineal resection (APR), the treatment portal must be extended to cover the perineum and surgical scar.

Portal design depends on the location of the primary tumor, risk of adjacent nodal involvement, and presence of adjacent organ involvement. However, the following generalizations are commonly employed in treatment portal arrangement.

Both four field and three field (posterior and two laterals) treatment ports have been used successfully. The 3 field is commonly used and will be described here:

Patients are treated in the prone position so that the lateral ports can adequately encompass the posterior portion of the sacrum.

For patients receiving postoperative radiation, oral contrast may be given several hours prior to simulation in order to assess the amount of small bowel in the treatment portal. Both surgical and radiation techniques have been utilized to reduce the amount of small bowel in the treatment volume. These methods include pelvic reconstruction with reperitonealization, treating the patient prone with bladder distension, or a special small bowel displacement board used to allow the bowel to fall away from the pelvis.

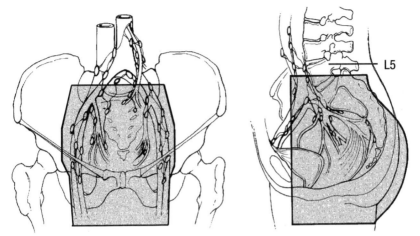

Fig. 6.13 PA and Lateral Treatment Ports for Rectal Cancer
Following Low Anterior Resection

PA Field Borders:

Superior: bottom of L5
Inferior: at least 5 cm below the tumor (may need to
include the anal margin for low rectal tumors)
Lateral: 1-2 cm beyond the pelvic inlet

Lateral Field Borders:

Posterior: posterior to the sacrum
Anterior: anterior to or mid-acetabulum (inclusion of the
vagina is necessary in the female patient)

Following APR, it is important to include the perineum in
the treatment portal in order to decrease the risk of a
perineal recurrence secondary to tumor implantation at the
time of surgery. The perineal scar is usually marked with a
radiopaque marker at the time of simulation.

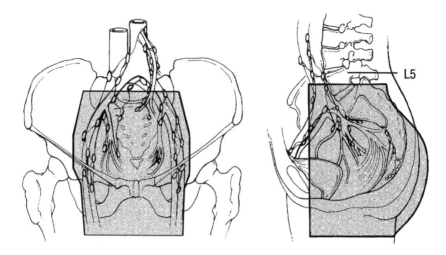

Fig. 6.14 PA and Lateral Treatment Ports following APR

PA Field Borders:

Superior: bottom of L5
Inferior: 1-2 cm below the perineal scar
Lateral: 1-2 cm beyond the pelvic inlet
NOTE: when treating the posterior port the scar should be bolused.

Lateral Field Borders:

Posterior: 1-2 cm beyond the perineal scar
Anterior: anterior to or mid-acetabulum

CT ANATOMY

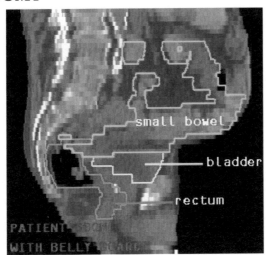

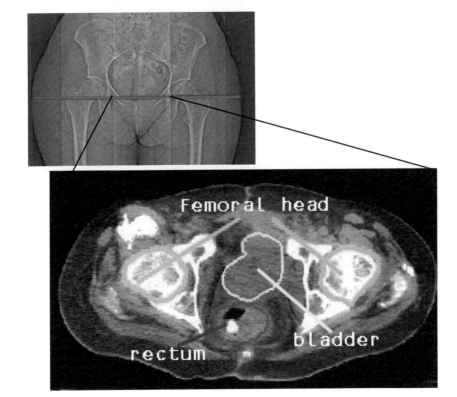

TOLERANCE DOSES

Critical Structure	Suggested Maximum Tolerance
Small Bowel	No more than 200 cc above 30 Gy
	No more than 150 cc above 35 Gy
	No more than 20 cc above 45 Gy
	None above 50 Gy
Femoral Heads	No more than 50% above 30 Gy
	No more than 35% above 40 Gy
	No more than 5% above 44 Gy
Iliac Crests	No more than 50% above 30 Gy
	No more than 35% above 40 Gy
	No more than 5% above 50 Gy
External Genitalia	No more than 50% above 20 Gy
	No more than 35% above 30 Gy
	No more than 5% above 40 Gy
Bladder	No more than 50% above 35 Gy
	No more than 35% above 40 Gy
	No more than 5% above 50 Gy
Large Bowel	No more than 200 cc above 30 Gy
	No more than 150 cc above 35 Gy
	No more than 20 cc above 45 Gy

Doses

45-50 Gy at 1.8 Gy per fraction is recommended.
After 45 Gy, a tumor bed boost of 5.4 Gy at 1.8 Gy per fraction (50.4 Gy total) can be considered for pre-operative radiation, and 5.4-9.0 Gy at 1.8 Gy per fraction (50.4-61.2 Gy total) for post-operative radiation.

ANUS

Cancers of the anal region are uncommon in comparison to other bowel tumors and are predominantly squamous cell carcinomas. Anal carcinomas have been associated with condylomas or genital warts, anal intercourse in men, genital infections, and other causes of chronic irritation.

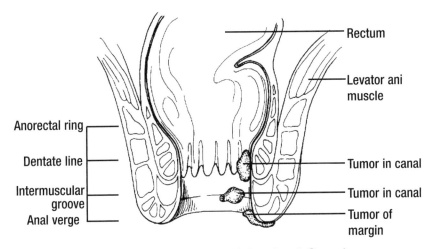

Fig. 6.15 Anatomy of the Anal Canal

The anal canal measures approximately 3 cm in length and extends from the anorectal ring superiorly to the anal verge inferiorly. The anal margin is defined as an area 5-6 cm in size surrounding the anal verge.

Routes of Spread

Anal cancers can spread by direct extension, lymphatics or the bloodstream. Hematogenous spread at the time of diagnosis is rare. Direct extension of anal cancers can involve the sphincter muscles, rectal wall, perianal skin, vaginal septum, prostate gland, sacrum and coccyx. Lymphatic spread from anal carcinomas occurs via three pathways. Tumors of the anal margin, anal verge and lower anal canal spread to the inguinal nodes. Carcinomas of the anal canal may also spread upward to the external and internal iliac nodes of the pelvis. Tumors of the upper anal canal and transition zone between the rectum and the anus may travel to the inferior mesenteric nodes. Hematogenous metastases may occur to the liver and the lungs.

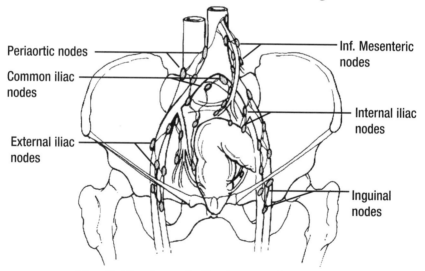

Fig. 6.16 Lymph Drainage of the Anus

Technical Aspects of Radiation Therapy

Historically, radical surgery, to include abdominoperineal resection, was the primary treatment for anal cancers. The use of combined radiation therapy and chemotherapy has resulted in a major treatment alternative in anal cancer and has improved survival, local control and sphincter preservation. Radical radiation therapy alone has also been used successfully especially with smaller tumors of the anus. Currently, most oncologists prefer treatment protocols using chemotherapy and radiation, reserving radical surgery for residual or recurrent disease.

Treatment portals are designed to include the primary tumor and regional nodes. Patients are simulated supine to allow visualization of the inguinal areas and a radiopaque marker is placed on the inferior most extension of the tumor or anal verge. A 3D conformal multiple field technique, or IMRT, to include volumetric modulated arc-therapy, can be used to treat anal carcinoma. IMRT can deliver a conformal dose while often sparing more critical normal tissue than conventional techniques. Of greatest concern are the small bowel for advanced anal cancers and the femoral head and neck.

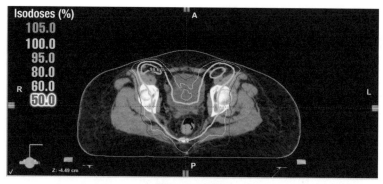

Fig. 6.17a

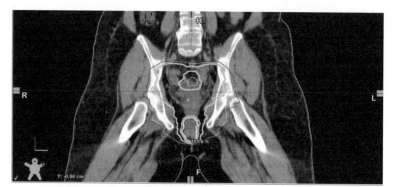

Fig. 6.17b

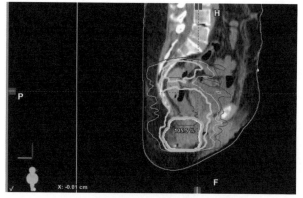

Fig. 6.17c

Volumetric Modulated Arc Therapy (VMAT) for Anal Cancer

Treatment Borders

Pelvic Field (PTV) – Anus, Perineum, Pelvic nodes: external iliac, internal iliac, pre-sacral, and inguinal nodes

Superior: L5-S1
Inferior: include the anus with a minimum of 2.5 cm margin around the anus and the tumor
Lateral: inclusion of the inguinal nodes

Lower Pelvic Field (CTV) – Anus, perineum, external iliac and inguinal nodes

Superior: bottom of sacroiliac (SI) joints
Inferior: include the anus with a minimum of 2.5 cm margin around the anus and the tumor
Lateral: inclusion of the inguinal nodes

Boost Field (GTV) - Primary tumor and involved nodes with a 2-2.5 cm margin

Doses

Recent studies suggest that the pelvic field (PTV) be treated to 30.6 Gy, the reduced pelvic field (CTV) should be treated to at least 45 Gy. This field could be further reduced off of the inguinal nodes at 36 Gy if inguinal nodes are negative. For large tumors or residual disease, the tumor and involved nodes (GTV) can be boosted to a total dose of 54-59 Gy at 1.8-2.0 Gy per fraction.

A simultaneous integrated boost (SIB) can deliver the required dose to the GTV and to the PTV in one process. A dose of 59.4 Gy to the gross disease (1.8 Gy per fraction) can be delivered at the same time that 49.5 Gy (1.5 Gy per fraction) is delivered to the subclinical disease. This method can be delivered with an IMRT or VMAT technique.

Chapter 7

Genitourinary Cancers

BLADDER

The majority of bladder cancers are diagnosed in the 50-60 year old population. Frequently, these tumors arise as superficial lesions without evidence of invasion into the muscular wall of the bladder. The most common presenting symptom is hematuria. Dysuria and frequent urination are also common complaints. Risk factors in the development of bladder cancer have been identified and include cigarette smoking, exposure to aniline dyes, and chronic bladder irritation.

Anatomy

The bladder is composed of a muscular wall with the two ureteral orifices located posterior and laterally. The urethral orifice is located at the base of the bladder. The triangular area between the three orifices is called the trigone of the bladder. This area is one of the most common sites for carcinoma.

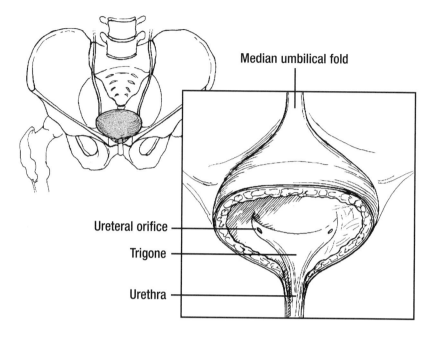

Fig. 7.1 Anatomy of the Bladder - Frontal Section

Routes of Spread

Carcinoma of the bladder can spread by direct extension into and through the bladder wall. If the cancer penetrates the mucosal surface of the bladder wall, spread through either the bloodstream or the lymphatics is possible. The primary route of lymphatic drainage is the external and internal iliac nodes.

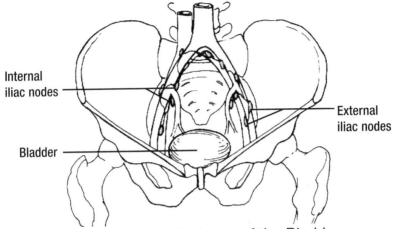

Fig. 7.2 Lymph Drainage of the Bladder

Treatment Options

Surgery is the treatment of choice for small, localized tumors of the bladder. Cancer that has not invaded the bladder wall can be successfully treated by a transurethral resection of the bladder (TURB). A partial cystectomy can be performed if the tumor is accessible and can be completely removed without compromising the bladder function. Invasive bladder cancers generally require a cystectomy to remove the entire bladder, as well as surrounding lymph nodes. A radical cystectomy typically includes the removal of the prostate and seminal vesicles in men, and the uterus, ovaries and part of the vagina in women. If the patient cannot tolerate a radical cystectomy, a partial cystectomy or a TURB may be followed by chemotherapy and radiation, or radiation alone if the chemotherapy cannot be tolerated. Low dose pre-operative radiation therapy has been used to downsize the tumor before surgery.

Technical Aspects of Radiation Therapy

A four field isocentric technique is often used when treating the bladder and regional lymph nodes. The patient should be simulated and treated with the bladder empty.

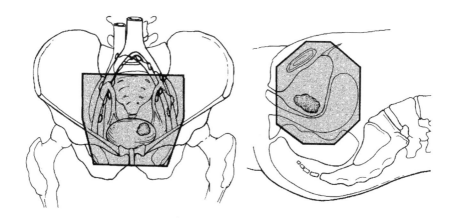

Fig. 7.3 AP-PA and Lateral Treatment Borders for Bladder Cancer

AP/PA borders are as follows:

Superior: between S1 and S2
Inferior: bottom of the obturator foramen
Lateral: one to two centimeters beyond the bony pelvic side walls. (Field shaping is usually done around the femurs).

Lateral Borders are as follows:

Anterior: usually extends 1-2 cm beyond the bladder (approximately 1-2 cm anterior to the pubic symphysis)
Posterior: usually extends 2-3 cm behind the bladder and tumor volume. Dose to surrounding normal tissue and to critical structures, such as the posterior rectal wall, small bowel and anus, should be limited.

If the patient is a candidate for definitive radiation therapy, careful planning of the boost portal is done with the use of a CT scan, physical exam, cystoscopy and a urologist's diagram of the tumor. Careful planning can alleviate the need to treat the entire bladder and decrease both acute and long term side effects. Boost portals should be simulated with a minimum of a 2 cm margin around the tumor volume. Techniques for boost treatments include parallel opposed or multiple conformal fields (e.g., AP-PA, lateral, or obliques).

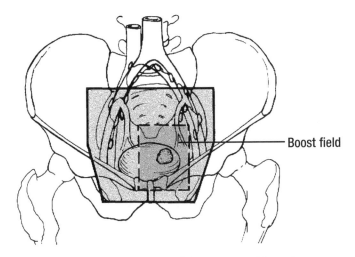

Fig. 7.4 Bladder Treatment Boost

Dose

Preoperative radiation therapy is usually given via a four field technique to include the entire bladder and regional lymph nodes. Preoperatively, patients receive a dose of 45-50 Gy at 1.8 Gy per fraction. Surgery is then performed in three weeks.

For patients not able to undergo surgery or receive chemo-therapy, definitive radiation therapy is an option. It is usually recommended that the patient have a transurethral resection of as much of the gross tumor as possible for best results. When primary radiation therapy is used to spare the bladder, opposed to a cystectomy, 40 Gy may be delivered, typically with a 4 field technique. If residual disease is found after 40 Gy, a cystectomy is recommended. If no disease is apparent, an additional 25 Gy may be delivered. Concurrent chemotherapy should be delivered per protocol specifications.

PROSTATE

Prostate cancer is the most common cancer in men. Almost half of all newly diagnosed prostate cancers are clinically localized, asymptomatic cancers. This increase in the diagnosis of early stage cancers is due to an increased use of prostate specific antigen (PSA) screening.

Patients may present with obstructive symptoms, an area of induration on rectal exam, or with an elevated PSA. PSA is an antigen found in seminal vesicle fluid and plasma which is produced by benign and malignant cells in the prostate. PSA is the best tumor marker for prostate cancer and is an important prognostic indicator. The level of PSA directly correlates with the patient's clinical stage, Gleason score, and treatment failure rate.

Routes of Spread

Prostate cancer may spread by local invasion, to involve the periprostatic tissue, seminal vesicles, bladder, and/or ureters. Prostate cancer can also spread through the lymphatic system. The first area of nodal spread is to the periprostatic and the obturator lymph nodes. Internal iliac, external iliac, common iliac, presciatic and presacral nodes may also be involved. Lymphatic spread increases with the stage and the grade of the tumor. Hematogenous metastases is seen with advanced disease. The most common metastatic site is bone.

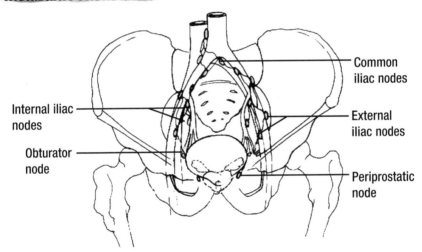

Fig. 7.5 Lymph Drainage of the Prostate

Anatomy

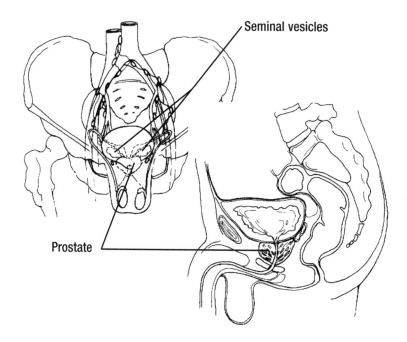

Fig.7.6 Anatomical Relations of the Prostate Gland

The prostate is attached anteriorly to the pubic symphysis. Superior to the prostate are the seminal vesicles and the bladder. The rectum is posterior to the prostate. Lateral to the prostate is the levater-ani muscle. The urogenital diaphragm is inferior to the prostate. The prostate gland is composed of five lobes. It consists of an anterior, a posterior, a medial and two lateral lobes. The urethra passes through the prostate gland.

The demarcation of the anatomical position of the prostate in relation to the bladder, rectum, and bony structures of the pelvis is critical in external beam treatment planning. The position of the prostate may vary in each patient.

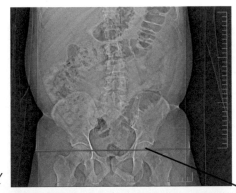

CT ANATOMY

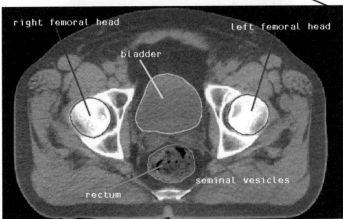

MR ANATOMY

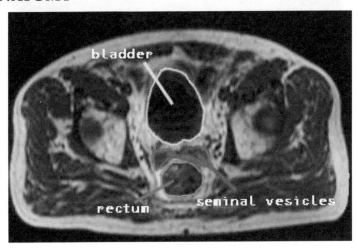

CT and MR ANATOMY *(MR diagram on next page)*

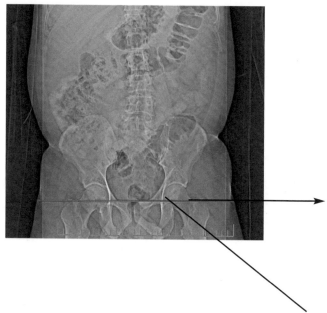

CT ANATOMY

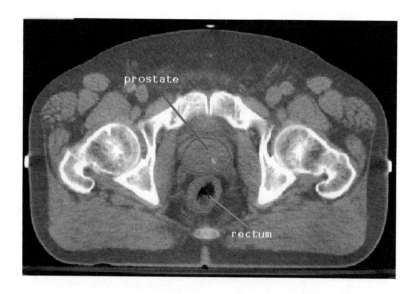

MR ANATOMY

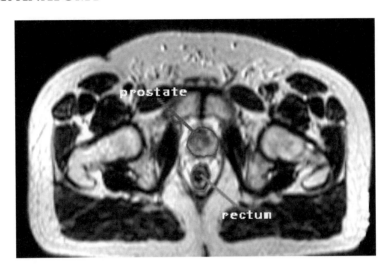

TOLERANCE DOSES

Suggested Tolerance Doses for Organs Surrounding the Prostate

Critical Structure	Suggested Maximum Tolerance
Rectum	No more than 55% above 47 Gy
	No more than 30% above 65 Gy
	None above 82 Gy
Bladder	No more than 55% above 47 Gy
	No more than 40% above 65 Gy
	No more than 25% above 70 Gy
	None above 82 Gy
Femoral Heads	No more than 50% above 30 Gy
	No more than 35% above 40 Gy
	No more than 5% above 44 Gy

Treatment

Current recommendations for treatment of early stage prostate cancers include: active surveillance, radical prostatectomy or radiation therapy. The treatment of choice is influenced by the patient's age, general health status, tumor aggressiveness, potential side effects of treatment and patient preference.

Technical Aspects of Radiation Therapy

IMRT with image guidance is a standard treatment technique for prostate cancer. The anatomical position of the prostate gland and seminal vesicles in relation to the bladder, rectum and bony structures of the pelvis can be outlined using a treatment planning CT. The CT can be fused with an MRI to assist in identifying the apex (lower portion) of the prostate, as well as muscular borders. 3-dimensional planning reduces the risk of acute toxicities and allows for the accurate administration of higher doses of radiation to the target volume.

The prostate should be localized daily prior to definitive radiation treatment. Some common methods to localize the prostate include: cone beam CT, ultrasound, implanted fiducials, and electromagnetic tracking. Based upon defined prognostic indicators, treatment volumes may include the prostate gland with or without seminal vesicles, and the regional lymph nodes for high risk cases. Brachytherapy is an option for early stage cancers, or can be combined with external beam radiation therapy (EBRT) for intermediate or high risk cancers. Patients with very large or very small prostate glands are not good candidates for brachytherapy. Androgen Deprivation Therapy (ADT) can be used to shrink the prostate prior to brachytherapy.

Radiation can be administered following a prostatectomy and is indicated for patients with a high risk for recurrence. Patients with positive surgical margins, seminal vesicle involvement, large tumors, or those with rising PSA or high Gleason scores, and without metastatic disease are generally considered candidates for radiation to the prostate bed. Regional lymph nodes may be included in the targeted volume. When regional lymph nodes are included with the treatment to the prostate, or the prostate bed, a simultaneous integrated boost technique can be employed. The regional lymph nodes usually receive 45-50 Gy while the prostate bed or prostate gland can be boosted to the recommended prescribed doses.

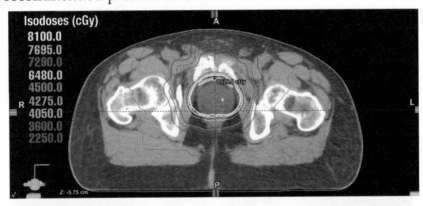

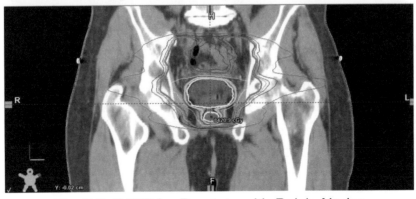

Fig. 7.7 IMRT for Prostate with Pelvic Nodes

Dose

A dose of 75.6-79.2 Gy at 1.8 -2.0 Gy/fraction (standard fractionation) to the prostate (with or without the seminal vesicles to a dose of 45-50 Gy) is recommended for low risk.

Intermediate and high risk receive doses up to 81 Gy to the prostate using standard fractionation. Patients with high risk cancers are candidates for pelvic node irradiation (to 45-50 Gy) and ADT. Trials are ongoing to evaluate hypofractionated schemes.   45 Gy is delivered to the prostate, seminal vesicles, and lymph nodes, with a simultaneous integrated boost to the prostate alone, to a total dose of 67.5 Gy in 25 fractions.

A dose of 45-50 Gy to the prostate (with or without the seminal vesicles) is recommended when combined with a brachytherapy boost to the prostate.

64-68 Gy in 1.8-2.0 Gy/fraction is currently recommended for post-operative radiation to the prostate bed.

TESTICULAR CANCER

Survival rates of testicular cancers have improved over the past twenty years, primarily due to advances in chemotherapy. All stages considered, the overall survival rate for cancer of the testis is 80%. Although testicular cancer accounts for less than 2% of all cancers in males, it is the most common malignancy in young men between the ages of 15-34. Testicular tumors usually present as a painless swelling in one gonad and are often detected by self-palpation. Because 95% of all testicular neoplasms arise from germ cells and the majority are seminomas, we have limited the following discussion to seminomas.

Anatomy

During the development of the fetus, the testicles form near the second lumbar vertebra. As their development continues, the testicles descend into the scrotal sac. The blood vessels and lymphatics follow the testicles from the lumbar region into the scrotal sac. There is an increased incidence of testicular neoplasms in patients with undescended testes. It is thought that these tumors are related to gonadal dysgenesis.

Routes of Spread

Pure seminomas, when detected early, are often localized to the scrotum. The primary route of spread is through the lymphatics. Due to the site of origin of the testis, the lymph nodes that are most commonly involved are the periaortic nodes along the lumbar vertebra and below the kidneys. On the left side, the primary nodes involved are the periaortic nodes below the renal vein. On the right side, the primary nodes are the lymphatics along the inferior vena cava. There can be cross-over drainage between these two groups of nodes. Therefore, both groups of nodes are at risk. In the pelvic area, some of the draining lymphatics terminate in the iliac nodes. Generally, only the lymphatics on the effected side are involved, unless there is a history of the patient having surgery in the groin or the pelvis which could alter the normal lymphatic flow. From the periaortic nodes there is usually an orderly spread to either the mediastinal nodes or the left supraclavicular nodes by way of the thoracic duct.

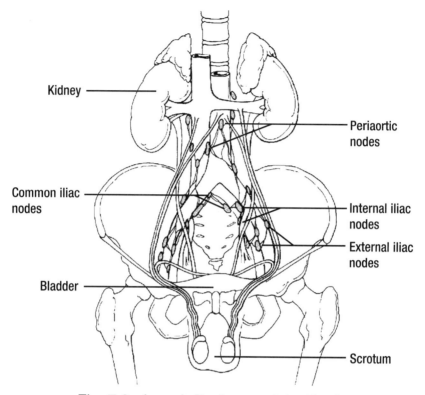

Kidney

Periaortic nodes

Common iliac nodes

Internal iliac nodes

External iliac nodes

Bladder

Scrotum

Fig. 7.8   Lymph Drainage of the Testis

Treatment Options

The initial treatment for most patients who present with a testicular mass is an inguinal orchiectomy. For early stage (IA or IB) seminoma, treatment options following the orchiectomy include: surveillance, radiation therapy or chemotherapy. The overall survival rate for early stage is 99% regardless of the treatment chosen. Chemotherapy is considered equally as effective as radiation therapy, and potentially less toxic. Surveillance involves close follow up. The most common site of relapse following surveillance or chemotherapy is the retroperitoneal nodes.

When radiation is chosen to treat early stage seminomas, with no history of pelvic or scrotal surgery, the current recommendation is to treat periaortic fields only. For patients who have had pelvic surgery, the lymphatic drainage of the testis may have been altered. Radiation therapy portals should include the ipsilateral pelvic nodes and the surgical scar.

Radiation therapy has been the primary treatment following orchiectomy for Stage IIA and IIB seminomas. The radiation field generally includes the periaortic and ipsilateral iliac field. Overall survival for this stage is 99%. For Stage IIB patients with lymph nodes greater than 3 cm, chemotherapy may be recommended opposed to radiation therapy.

For later stage IIC and III seminomas, chemotherapy is currently the treatment of choice.

Technical Aspects of Radiation Therapy

Lymph nodes included in the periaortic field are: periaortic, paracaval, interaortocaval and preaortic nodes.

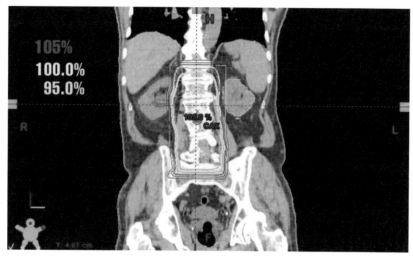

Fig. 7.9

Borders for a Periaortic Field:

Superior: bottom of T-11
Inferior: bottom of L-5
Lateral borders: approximately 10 cm wide encompassing the tips of the transverse processes of the periaortic vertebrae.

Critical Structure	Suggested Maximum Tolerance
Kidneys	No more than 50% of each kidney above 8 Gy
	If only one kidney, No more than 15% above 20 Gy

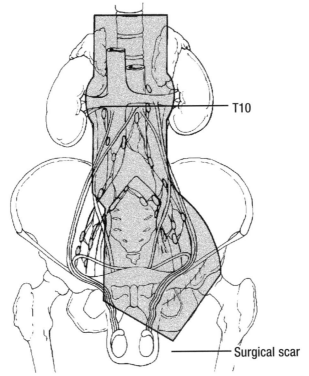

Fig. 7.10 Hockey Stick (or Dog Leg) Treatment Field
for Testicular Cancer

Borders for the Hockey Stick (Dog Leg) Field:

The lymph nodes to be included are: periaortic, paracaval,
interaortocaval and preaortic nodes, and the ipsilateral
common, external, and proximal internal iliac nodes down
to the top of the acetabulum.

Superior: at the bottom of T-11
Inferior: top of acetabulum
Lateral: (periaortic region) approximately 10 cm wide
encompassing the transverse processes of the
vertebral bodies

Lateral: (pelvic region) edge of the ilium to include the ipsilateral iliac nodes. The ipsilateral inguinal area and the surgical scar may be included.

Medial: (pelvic region) approximately midline to encompass the ipsilateral common, external and proximal internal iliac nodes with at least a 1.2 cm margin to account for setup error and patient motion. In standard cases, a line can be drawn from the contralateral transverse process of the fifth lumbar vertebrae to the medial border of the ipsilateral obturator foramen.

Dose

Periaortic Fields (Stage I) - 20 Gy in 2 Gy per fraction
Hockey Stick Fields (Stage II) – 20 Gy in 2 Gy per fraction or 25.5 Gy in 1.7 Gy per fraction

If required, a nodal mass boost should include the gross tumor volume with a 2 cm margin, treated with AP-PA fields. 30-36 Gy is delivered in 2 Gy per fraction.

Chapter 8

Gynecological Cancers

UTERINE CERVIX

With the advent of the pap smear, the incidence of invasive carcinoma of the cervix has decreased significantly. Cancer of the cervix is the third most common cancer in women worldwide. The majority of cases are found in developing countries, where the human papilloma virus (HPV) is more prevalent. Chronic HPV has been identified as a major risk factor for cervical cancer.

Anatomy

The uterus is located in the true pelvis, posterior to the bladder and anterior to the rectum. The three portions of the uterus are the fundus (superiorly), the corpus (body), and the cervix (inferiorly).

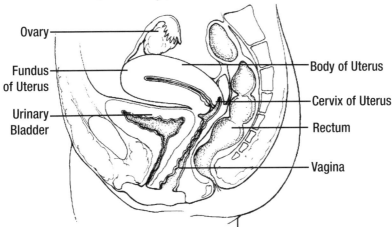

Fig. 8.1 Lateral View of Female Pelvis

MR FEMALE PELVIS (LATERAL VIEW)

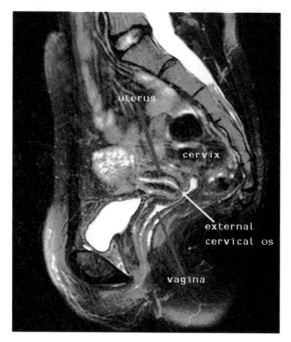

Routes of Spread

Squamous cell cancer is the most common pathologic type of cancer of the cervix. The cancer usually begins at the endocervical canal, or at the external os (opening of the cervix). Initially, cervical cancer may grow downward into the lateral fornices (the superior most portion of the vagina). If the cancer extends superiorly, the lower uterine segment may be involved. The cancer may also extend anteriorly into the bladder, posteriorly into the rectum or laterally into the parametrium. The parametrium is composed of ligaments, connective tissues, blood vessels and lymph nodes that lie lateral to the cervix, and help support the uterus.

The cervix and uterus are fortified by a rich lymphatic system. The three most frequently involved group of nodes are the obturator, internal iliac and external iliac lymph nodes. The obturator nodes are a part of the external iliac chain and can be found against the pelvic wall, slightly above the acetabulum.

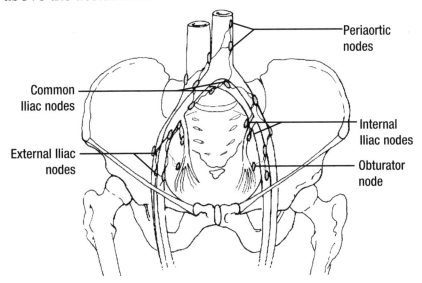

Fig. 8.2a Lymph Nodes of the Pelvis

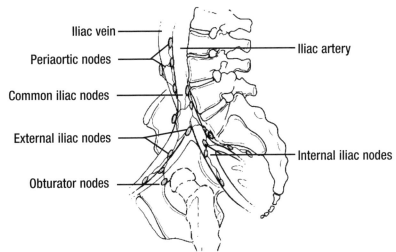

Fig. 8.2b Pelvic Lymph Nodes-Lateral View

The internal iliac, or hypogastric nodes begin at the bifurcation of the common iliac nodes and are located approximately 4-5 cm posterior to the obturator nodes. The common iliac and periaortic nodes are less frequently involved, but are at risk, especially with more advanced disease. The common iliac nodes extend from the top of L5 to the beginning of the internal iliac and external iliac chains, in the front of the sacrum.

Technical Aspects of Radiation Therapy

External beam is generally used in combination with intracavitary irradiation for cancer of the cervix. The role of external beam is to sterilize central disease and nodal disease that may lie outside the realm of intracavitary treatment. External beam is also used to help shrink bulky central disease to allow for optimal brachytherapy placement.

When designing the radiation ports, the known disease and potential sites of lymphatic spread must be encompassed.

At a minimum, the treatment volume should cover the gross disease, the parametria, the uterosacral ligaments, a sufficient vaginal margin from the gross disease (at least 3 cm), the presacral nodes and any other nodal volumes at risk. For patients with negative nodes, the radiation volume should include the external iliac, internal iliac, and the obturator nodes.

For bulkier tumors or positive nodes in the lower true pelvis, the radiation volume should be increased to cover the common iliac nodes as well.

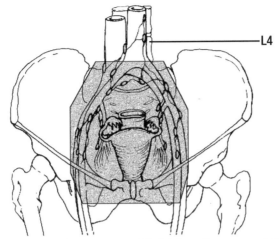

L4

Fig. 8.3a   AP-PA Treatment Field for Cancer of the Cervix

The AP-PA Portal is set up with the following borders:

Superior: L4-L5 interspace

Inferior: the bottom of the obturator foramen (A radio-paque vaginal cylinder may be used to delineate the cervix and to assure that the treatment port is 3-4 cm below the known disease)

Lateral: a minimum of 1 cm lateral to the pelvic brim to encompass the external and internal iliac nodes. The common iliac nodes lie medial to the sacroiliac (SI) joints; therefore, blocking may be used to exclude tissue lateral to the SI joints.

In patients with documented common iliac or periaortic involvement, extended field or periaortic radiation therapy is recommended, up to the level of the renal vessels or higher based on nodal involvement. IMRT and conformal fields can help limit the dose to the bowel and other critical structures.

Brachytherapy is often used to treat central disease for patients with an intact cervix. Brachytherapy can be the primary treatment for patients who are not candidates for surgery. When brachytherapy is combined with external beam radiation therapy , the intracavitary insertion is performed following external beam, or intermittently, to boost the dose to the central disease. Scheduling the brachytherapy after, or during the latter part of the course of external beam therapy, allows time for tumor regression, and can improve the ability to accurately place the applicator.

In post-hysterectomy patients with positive surgical margins, the upper 3-4 cm of the vaginal cuff, the parametria, and adjacent lymph nodes may be treated with external beam radiation. A brachytherapy boost may be utilized.

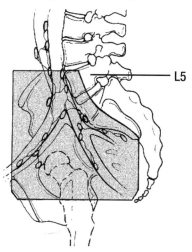

Fig. 8.3b Lateral Treatment Field for Cancer of the Cervix

If a lateral field is used the borders are as follows:

Anterior: encompassing the pubic symphysis
Posterior: split the sacrum. (Blocks may be added to reduce the rectal dose and the dose to the small bowel).

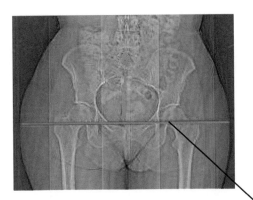

CT ANATOMY

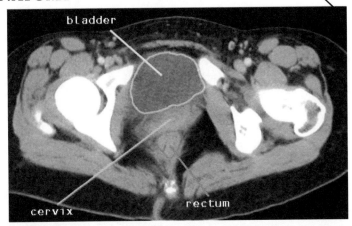

MR ANATOMY

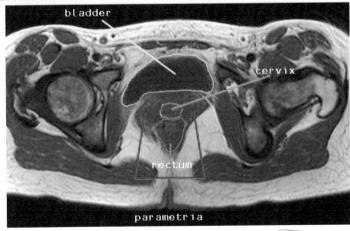

TOLERANCE DOSES

Critical Structure	Suggested Maximum Tolerance
Rectum	No more than 55% above 47 Gy
	No more than 30% above 65 Gy
	None above 82 Gy
Bladder	No more than 55% above 47 Gy
	No more than 40% above 65 Gy
	No more than 25% above 70 Gy
	None above 82 Gy
Femoral Heads	No more than 50% above 30 Gy
	No more than 35% above 40 Gy
	No more than 5% above 44 Gy

Suggested Tolerance Doses for Critical Structures near the Periaotic fields		
Organ	Suggested Tolerance	Endpoint
Spinal Cord	Max ≤45 Gy	Myelitis/Necrosis
Kidneys	Mean dose to bilateral kidneys should be 18 Gy. If patient has only one kidney, not more than 15% should receive ≥ 18 Gy and no more than 30% ≥ 14 Gy	Renal insufficiency

Dose

When radiation is the primary treatment, the tumor and the regional lymphatics at risk are typically treated to 45-50 Gy at 1.8-2.0 Gy/day. The primary tumor can be boosted with intracavitary brachytherapy to doses of 80-85 Gy to Point A. The majority of patients receive concurrent chemotherapy with radiation.

Limited volumes of gross disease outside of the cervix can be boosted using external beam therapy to total doses of 55-65 Gy.

ENDOMETRIUM

Carcinoma of the endometrium is the most common malignant lesion that arises from the female genital tract. The uterine cavity is made up of a mucous membrane lining (endometrium), a smooth muscle layer (myometrium), and an outer serous coat (peritoneum).

Routes of Spread

Most endometrial cancers are confined to the uterus initially. Spread of endometrial cancer is contiguous and involves the muscular wall. Once the smooth muscle has been penetrated, the incidence of lymph node involvement increases. The lymphatics that are commonly involved include the external iliac, the internal iliac, the common iliac, and the periaortic nodes. Transperitoneal spread may occur in endometrial cancer, as in ovarian cancer, and generally indicates more advanced disease.

Direct extension may occur and involve the cervix, vagina, bladder, and rectum.

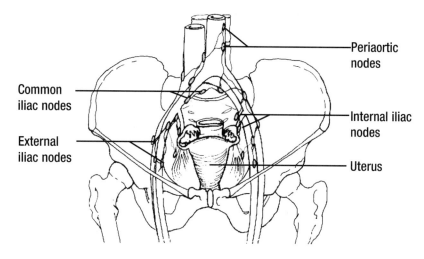

Common
iliac nodes

External
iliac nodes

Periaortic
nodes

Internal iliac
nodes

Uterus

Fig. 8.4 Lymph Drainage of the Uterus

Technical Aspects of Radiation Therapy

Both preoperative and postoperative external beam
irradiation and brachytherapy have been used in the
treatment of endometrial cancer. Most oncologists in the
United States prefer post-op radiation therapy, depending
on the extent of tumor pathologically. Radiation therapy is
recommended when the tumor extends beyond the inner
one-half of the myometrium or when tumor extends
beyond the uterus.

External beam treatment generally consists of conformal
whole pelvis ports.

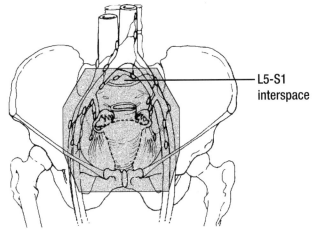

Fig. 8.5a AP-PA Treatment Borders for Endometrial Cancer

Treatment field borders are as follows:

Superior: L5-S1 interspace, to include the common iliac nodes

Inferior: bottom of the obturator foramen or to include at least one-half of the vagina. (A radiopaque vaginal localizer is used to assure adequate coverage of the upper vagina).

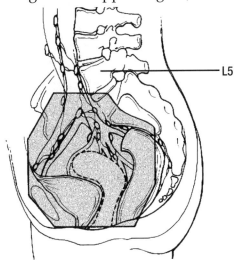

Fig. 8.5b Lateral Field Borders for Cancer of the Uterus

Borders for the lateral ports are as follows:

Anterior: encompassing the pubic symphysis

Posterior: split the sacrum. (Blocks may be added to reduce the rectal dose and the dose to the small bowel). In patients with periaortic involvement, extended field or periaortic radiation therapy is recommended, up to the level of the renal vessels or higher based on nodal involvement. IMRT and conformal fields can help limit the dose to the bowel and other critical structures.

CT and MR ANATOMY

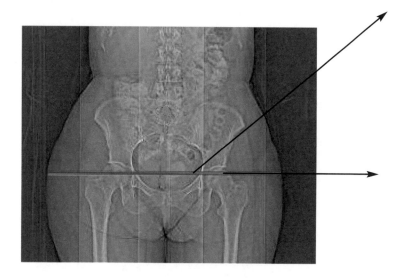

CT ANATOMY

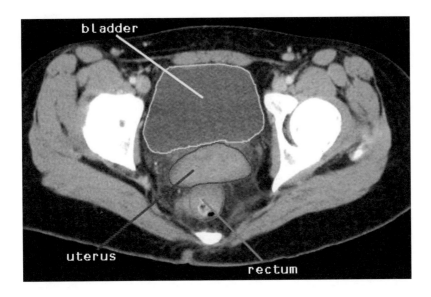

MR ANATOMY

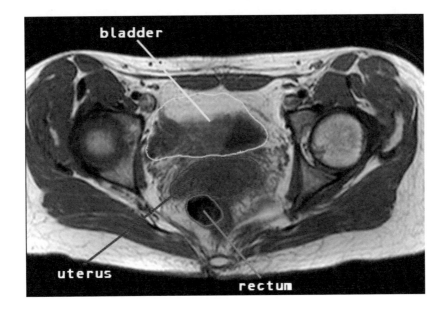

TOLERANCE DOSES

Critical Structure	Suggested Maximum Tolerance
Rectum	No more than 55% above 47 Gy
	No more than 30% above 65 Gy
	None above 82 Gy
Bladder	No more than 55% above 47 Gy
	No more than 40% above 65 Gy
	No more than 25% above 70 Gy
	None above 82 Gy
Femoral Heads	No more than 50% above 30 Gy
	No more than 35% above 40 Gy
	No more than 5% above 44 Gy

Suggested Tolerance Doses for Critical Structures near the Periaotic fields		
Organ	Suggested Tolerance	Endpoint
Spinal Cord	Max ≤45 Gy	Myelitis/Necrosis
Kidneys	Mean dose to bilateral kidneys should be 18 Gy. If patient has only one kidney, not more than 15% should receive ≥ 18 Gy and no more than 30% ≥ 14 Gy	Renal insufficiency

Dose

The pelvis is treated to a total of 45-50 Gy with 1.8-2.0 Gy per fraction. Brachytherapy may also be considered to the vaginal cuff.

Chapter 9

Pediatric Tumors

Major progress has been made in treatment techniques for pediatric oncology patients. Enrollment in protocols, combined with major advances in therapy, has resulted in a dramatic improvement in the survival and quality of life of these children.

Organs, bone and soft tissue are still developing in pediatric patients; therefore, late effects of aggressive therapy may be severe. Surgeons, medical oncologists, and radiation oncologists must make an effort to be conservative, without abandoning efforts to cure or control the tumor. For these reasons, pediatric patients should be enrolled on protocols in which the specific radiation doses and treatment portals are outlined. A multimodality approach is generally used to decrease side effects.

Typical treatment portals are presented in this chapter as a general guideline. It is important to consult current protocols for specific criteria.

ACUTE LEUKEMIA

Acute leukemia, a malignant disease of bone marrow, is the most common malignancy in children. Chemotherapy is the mainstay of treatment. The majority of patients will develop disease throughout the central nervous system (CNS). Children currently receive systemic chemotherapy along with some type of CNS prophylaxis, depending on the risk status of the disease. Options for CNS prophylaxis include CNS-pentrant chemotherapy or cranial irradiation. Spinal radiation is no longer used. Whole body irradiation may be used when performing a bone marrow transplant.

Anatomy

The central nervous system is surrounded by meninges which consist of the pia (innermost layer), the arachnoid and the dura mater. Cerebrospinal fluid flows inside of the subarachnoid space, which is the space between the arachnoid and the pia.

Routes of Spread

Acute lymphocytic leukemia is a disorder of stem cells and results from an overgrowth of immature lymphoid and myloid cells called "blasts" which replace bone marrow cells. Blast cells can infiltrate the periosteum, liver, lymph nodes, or spleen. The central nervous system is involved in approximately 3% of children at diagnosis. The CNS and testicles are "sanctuary sites" at risk for harboring disease. When the CNS is involved the entire subarachnoid space (any area cerebral spinal fluid flows) is at risk.

Technical Aspects of Radiation Therapy

Cranial irradiation combined with intrathecal methotrexate based chemotherapy is presently a treatment option to prevent relapse in high risk patients. For CNS therapy the target volume includes the entire subarachnoid space and optic nerves.

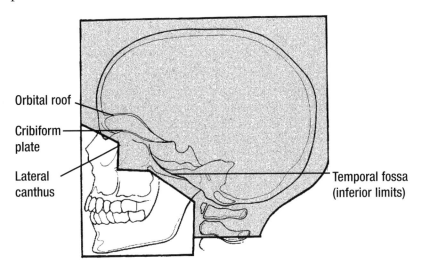

Fig. 9.1 Cranial Irradiation Field

The margins for the lateral cranial ports include:

Superior: fall off

Inferior: to include the cribiform plate and temporal fossa subfrontally; to the level of C2 posteriorly

Posterior: fall off (blocking can be added to spare tangential skin)

Anterior: fall off to cover the cranium

Proper attention to anatomical landmarks is imperative. Margins most likely to be inadequately covered include:

1) Cribiform plate - represents the inferior most site subfrontally and is sometimes difficult to include because of the proximity to the eyes.
2) Lower limit of the temporal fossa
3) Posterior retina and the optic nerve

To adequately encompass the posterior aspect of the retina and orbit while sparing the anterior half of the globe and lens, use a 4-5° gantry angle to correct for divergence.

CT ANATOMY

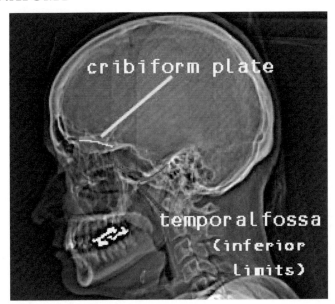

MR ANATOMY

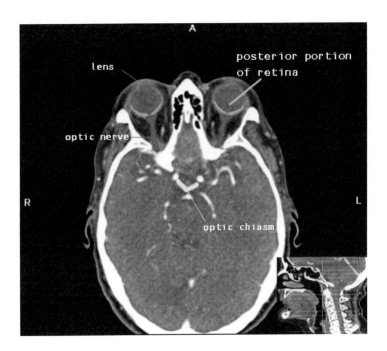

TOLERANCE DOSES

TD5/5 Normal Tissue Tolerances (Gy) 1.8–2.0 Gy/fraction				
Organ	1/3	2/3	3/3	End Point
Lens	10	10	10	Cataract
Lacrimal Gland	26	26	26	Dry eye
Optic Chiasm	50	50	50	Blindness
Optic Nerve	50	50	50	Blindness
Brain (temporal lobe)	58	51	47	Necrosis/Infarction
Brain Stem	60	53	50	Necrosis/Infarction
Spinal Cord	50 (5cm)	50 (10 cm)	47 (20 cm)	Myelitis/Necrosis
Ear	30	30	30	Acute serous otitis
Ear	55	55	55	Chronic serous otitis

Dose

There are ongoing trials to determine if radiation can be omitted from the treatment of children with ALL. The number of acute lymphocytic leukemia patients treated with radiation, and the total dose delivered, continue to decrease as less toxic chemotherapy regimens are discovered.

Most patients are treated on protocol, the current doses used for cranial irradiation are:
12-18 Gy at 1.8-2.0 Gy per fraction

MEDULLOBLASTOMA

Medulloblastoma is the most common malignant childhood brain tumor. Medulloblastomas comprise 18% of all pediatric tumors. The peak age for medulloblastoma is five years old. This tumor of neuroectodermal origin arises in the posterior fossa, principally in the midline of cerebellum.

Boundaries of the Posterior Fossa

The posterior fossa has the following boundaries:

Anterior: posterior clinoid
Superior: apex of the tentorium cerebelli (which is located half way between the foramen magnum and the vertex)
Posterior: posterior cranium
Inferior: occipital bone
Lateral: temporal, occipital, parietal bones

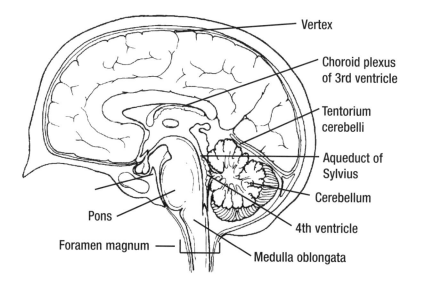

Fig. 9.2a

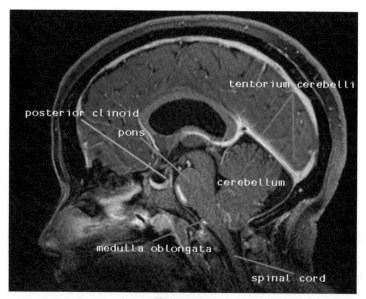

Fig. 9.2b

Routes of Spread

Medulloblastomas infiltrate locally and disseminate throughout the neuroaxis. About 45% have spread beyond the posterior fossa at presentation. These tumors can grow into and fill the fourth ventricle or involve the brain stem. They can extend supratentorially into the third ventricle or midbrain, or extend inferiorly to the upper cervical cord. Another major route of spread for medulloblastomas is dissemination throughout the ventricular system and the cerebrospinal fluid (CSF) pathways. Microscopic tumor cells are often found in the CSF, while gross nodular seeding may be present in the third or lateral ventricles, cerebral subarachnoid space, or spinal subarachnoid space. Medulloblastomas also metastasize systemically in 6% of the patients.

Technical Aspects of Radiation Therapy

Surgery is used initially for tissue diagnosis, tumor debulking and decompression. The goal of surgery is maximum tumor removal. Surgery alone is not curative due to the tendency of medulloblastomas to seed through the CSF. Treatment recommendations are based on the patient's age and risk stratification. In young patients, who are younger than 3 years old and sometimes as old as five years old, chemotherapy has been used to delay or replace radiation therapy. Postoperative craniospinal irradiation with adjuvant chemotherapy is recommended for all other patients.

When designing radiation portals, complete coverage of the subarachnoid space is imperative for irradiation of all CSF pathways. The head is treated through two lateral ports and the spine is treated through one posterior port. Most patients are treated in the prone position to facilitate daily setup at the junction over the cervical spine. A board can be used to elevate the patient's chest and abdomen and their forehead is placed on a headrest to align the cervical and thoracic spin. Maximum chin extension should be achieved to diminish exit radiation through the mandible when treating the spine field. The collimator for the lateral head fields should be angled to match the divergence of the spinal field. The treatment couch may also be angled to eliminate overlap from the divergence of the lateral head ports. The gaps between the cranial and spinal port should be moved two or three times throughout the treatment to prevent under or over dosage at the junction site. The field borders should be changed by increasing or decreasing the field borders the field lengths without changing the central ray.

The borders for the cranial port are as follows:

Superior: fall off

Inferior: to include the cribiform plate and temporal fossa subfrontally; to the level of C2 posteriorly

Posterior: fall off (blocking can be added to spare tangential skin posteriorly. However, this would be contraindicated with a menigocele)

Anterior: fall off to cover the cranium

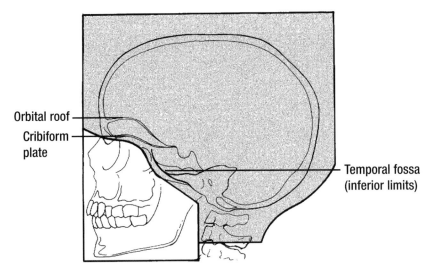

Orbital roof

Cribiform plate

Temporal fossa (inferior limits)

Fig. 9.3a Cranial Treatment Field

Spinal port:

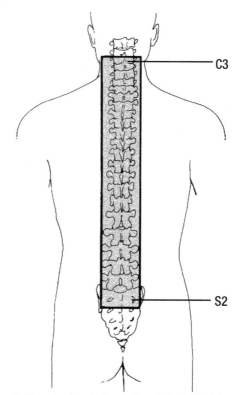

C3

S2

Fig. 9.3b Spinal Port for Medulloblastoma

Superior: junction of inferior border of the whole brain port
Inferior: below S2
Lateral: entire vertebral bodies with 1.0 cm margin
          (a spade portal is optional, but is not routinely
          done because sacral nerve involvement is rare)

The entire width of the vertebral bodies is included to cover
the width of the spinal cord and the CSF pathways; and
also to permit symmetrical growth after radiation.

Cranial Boost Field:
The cranial boost field encompasses the entire cerebellum, pons and medulla, extending from the tentorium to the foramen magnum.

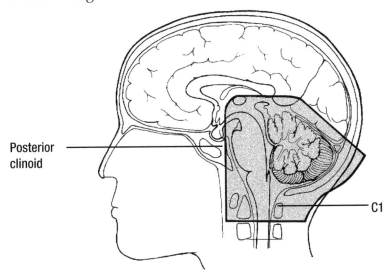

Posterior clinoid

C1

Fig. 9.3c Cranial Boost Port for Medulloblastoma

Superior: midway between foramen magnum and vertex, plus 1.0 cm
Inferior: bottom of C1
Anterior: posterior clinoid (attachment of the tentorium)
Posterior: behind calvarium

Dose

Most patients are treated on protocol. Patients may receive 36 Gy at 1.8 Gy per fraction to the whole brain and spine. Lower doses of 23.4 Gy are being studied with hopes to decrease long term neurocognitive effects. The posterior fossa, or tumor bed, is usually boosted to 54 Gy at 1.8 Gy per fraction. Adjuvant chemotherapy is a standard protocol recommendation.

EPENDYMOMA

Ependymomas occur in all age groups, but are most commonly found in children. In the adult, one-half of these tumors are infratentorial; whereas in children, two-thirds are infratentorial. Ependymomas represent about 6-10% of intracranial tumors in children and are more commonly seen in males.

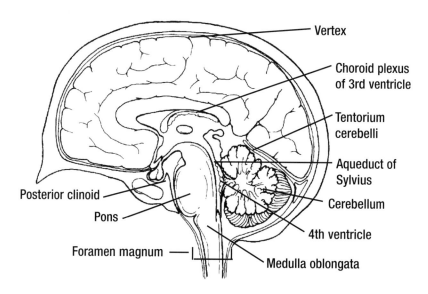

Fig. 9.4 Boundaries of the Posterior Fossa

Anatomy

Ependymomas arise from the ependymal lining of the ventricular system and spinal canal. Infratentorial ependymomas most commonly arise from the fourth ventricle.

Routes of Spread

Fourth ventricle ependymomas tend to spread locally, filling the fourth ventricle, or invading the cerebellum. They can also extend superiorly through the foramina of the fourth ventricle, or inferiorly through the foramen magnum to invade the upper cervical spine. One-third of the ependymomas arising from the fourth ventricle will extend beyond the foramen magnum. Careful attention must be given to the lower border of the posterior fossa portal, so that tumor is not excluded.

Ependymomas have been reported to seed the CSF (with an overall incidence of approximately 12%). CSF seeding is more commonly seen in high grade posterior fossa ependymomas. Presently, it has been shown that only 4% of patients with primary tumor control will seed through the CSF.

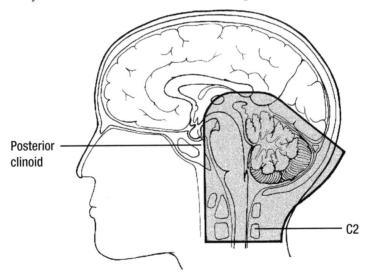

Fig. 9.5 Treatment Port for 4th Ventricle Ependymoma

Anterior: posterior clinoid
Superior: midway between foramen magnum and vertex plus one centimeter
Posterior: behind the calvarium
Inferior: C2-C3 interspace (with tumors that extend below the foramen magnum the lower border should be two vertebral levels below the preoperative tumor extent to a dose of 45 Gy)

Ependymomas are sensitive to chemotherapy, which has been used in some trials, but no definite benefit has been shown.

Technical Aspects of Radiation Therapy

Surgery is the first mode of treatment, with maximal tumor removal and preservation of neurologic function being the goal. Complete tumor removal is difficult because of the infiltrative nature of this tumor.

All patients greater than 3 years old are treated with postoperative radiation therapy. If the patient's spinal MRI or CSF cytology is positive for tumor, they should be treated with primary craniospinal irradiation (for portals see medulloblastoma section). Spinal dissemination is low in patients with negative CSF and no diagnostic findings. Conformal radiation to the tumor site alone is advocated and is proven to reduce the risk of recurrence at the site of origin.

Dose

The posterior fossa is standardly treated to 50-55.8 Gy at 1.8 Gy per fraction in children who are older than 3 years old.

When treating craniospinal portals, the standard dose is 36 Gy at 1.6-1.8 Gy per fraction. The gaps between the cranial and spinal port should be moved two to three times throughout the treatment to prevent under or overdosage at the junction site. The posterior fossa should be boosted to a total dose of 54-55.8 Gy.

BRAIN STEM GLIOMA

Brain stem gliomas occur in all age groups, but are often found in children. These tumors comprise 10-15% of all pediatric brain tumors. Histopathologically, brain stem gliomas range from low grade astrocytomas to high grade glioblastoma multiforme. 38% present as high grade tumors, and an additional 10% are ependymomas and primitive neuroectodermal tumors. The most common presenting symptom is gait disturbance. Patients may also present with a headache, hemiparesis, strabismus, or cranial nerve dysfunction.

Anatomy

Brain stem gliomas include tumors of the midbrain, pons, and medulla oblongata. 50% of brain stem gliomas arise in the pons. The brain stem is a complex structure comprising multiple cranial nerves and long tracts. The most common cranial nerve abnormalities demonstrated are the involvement of cranial nerves VI and VII. The pons and medulla lie against the clivus with the junction of the cervical cord and medulla being located radiographically at C1.

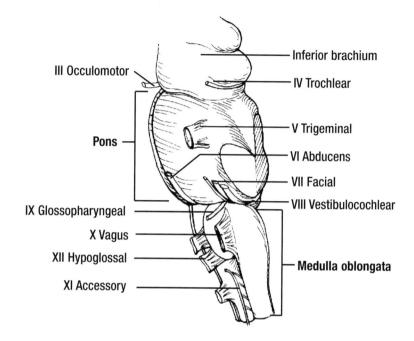

Fig. 9.6 The Brainstem

Routes of Spread

Brain stem gliomas infiltrate locally to involve the midbrain, pons, medulla, brachium pontis or cerebellum. Subarachnoid spread has been documented in 15-20% of children. The more anaplastic lesions will have more extensive local invasion and are more likely to disseminate.

Technical Aspects of Radiation Therapy

Because of the location and infiltrative nature of these tumors, they are not usually surgically resected. However, surgery is indicated in exophytic tumors with extension into the fourth ventricle which have little brain stem infiltration, tumors of the cervicomedullary junction, or tumors with a cystic component. Biopsy is generally not recommended, unless surgical resection is planned. Overall, the standard of treatment for brain stem gliomas is radiation therapy. Even though 15-20% spread through the CSF, a local field is the recommended treatment volume since most patients fail locally. Chemotherapy has also been used concomitantly in trials.

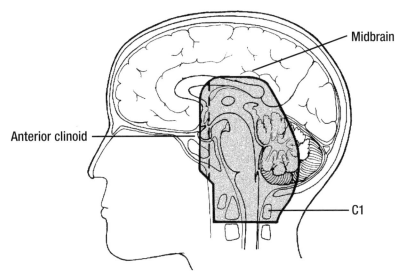

Fig. 9.7 Treatment Port for Tumor of the Pons

Treatment portal for a tumor of the pons:

Anterior: anterior clinoid
Note: Be careful to avoid the optic chiasm which usually lies anterior to the sella turcica. The anterior border may be placed at the "dotted" line as long as there is adequate margin around the tumor.
Superior: midbrain
Inferior: cervicomedullary junction (bottom of C1)
Posterior: mid-cerebellum

Important: The borders listed above are general borders that may need to be enlarged. An adequate margin must be placed on all areas of the tumor extension, as seen on MRI.

For midbrain tumors the entire extent of the tumor and a 1-2 cm margin are included in the treatment field.

Dose

Conventional doses range from 54-60 Gy at 1.5-2.0 Gy per fraction. Hyperfractionated (twice daily) treatments have been used to deliver higher doses ranging from 72-78 Gy in 1.0 Gy per fraction twice a day. To date, this technique has shown no survival benefit.

RHABDOMYOSARCOMA

Rhabdomyosarcoma is the most common soft tissue sarcoma of childhood. The peak incidence is between two and five years of age, with a second peak in incidence in adolescents between the ages of 15 and 19. Rhabdomyosarcoma has been associated with various syndromes (neurofibromatosis, Li-Fraumeni syndrome), environmental factors, and anomalies. Two-thirds of rhabdomyosarcoma patients will be long term survivors.

Anatomy

Rhabdomyosarcomas are malignant neoplasms derived from embryonic mesenchymal cells. They may occur at any location in the body. Histologic subtypes include embryonal, alveolar, pleomorphic and mixed variants. The embroyonal subtype accounts for approximately 60% of all cases. This subtype is most commonly found in the younger age group, and generally arises in the head and neck, or in genitourinary areas. The orbit is the most common site in the head and neck area. The alveolar subtype is more rare, accounting for approximately 20% of all cases. This subtype is more common in older children and generally presents in the extremities and perineal sites. It tends to metastasize through the lymphatics and overall has a poor prognosis. The pleomorphic and mixed variant subtypes are rare.

Routes of Spread

Rhabdomyosarcomas can spread by local extension, through the bloodstream, or the lymphatics. The lung, bone, bone marrow and lymph nodes are the most common sites of metastases. The incidence of lymph node metastases is dependent on the site of origin. The most common sites with positive lymph node metastases include the lower extremity (50%), and the paratesticular region (40%). Parameningeal tumors usually spread by intracranial extension, and invasion of the base of the skull is common. Lymph node involvement with orbital tumors is rare.

Technical Aspects of Radiation Therapy

Multimodality therapy, including tumor excision and organ preservation, is presently recommended. The amount of residual disease is a prognostic factor. Total excision of the tumor is preferred to biopsy alone, depending on the site. After surgical staging, all patients receive multiagent chemotherapy.

The radiation therapy portals will depend on the site and extent of the disease. Overall, the recommended volume for treatment includes the extent of the primary tumor and an adequate margin to cover the tumor and suspected areas of involvement. Generally, this is at least a 2-4 cm margin in length, and axially the margin should encompass the involved fascial plane.

If there is regional nodal involvement at diagnosis, the lymph node chain draining the regional area is included.

Normal tissue tolerance shall be taken into account in all patients.

A parameningeal location includes involvement of the middle ear, nasal cavity, nasopharynx, paranasal sinuses or infratemporal fossa. Irradiation of this area requires careful planning. Because of its uniqueness, a treatment volume for a parameningeal nasopharynx presentation will be illustrated (Fig. 9.8).

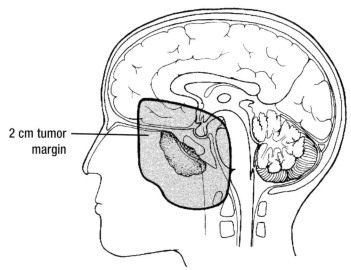

2 cm tumor margin

Fig. 9.8 Treatment Field for a Parameningeal Site

A 2 cm margin is included around the primary tumor and the base of the skull. Regional lymph nodes do not need to be included unless they are positive.

If intracranial meningeal extension is present in continuity with the primary tumor, a 2 cm margin is placed on the intracranial disease also (whole brain treatment is not necessary).

For a separate brain metastases the whole brain should be treated. If the CSF is positive, either craniospinal or whole brain irradiation and intrathecal methotrexate is utilized.

Dose

Current protocols must be consulted. Combined therapies are generally employed. A dose of 45-50 Gy may be used to shrink a tumor preoperatively. A 10-20 Gy boost postoperatively if residual disease remains. Postoperative radiation to doses of 55-60 Gy may be used when unresectable gross disease remains. All doses are dependent on the treatment regimen, the type, the location, and the extent of disease.

EWING'S SARCOMA

Ewing's sarcoma is the second most common bone tumor of childhood. It occurs more often in males (1.5:1) and is extremely rare in black children. A peak incidence is seen in the 10-15 year old age group. The most common site of involvement is the lower half of the body. It is frequently seen in the pelvic bones, femur, tibia, fibula, scapula, clavicles, ribs and vertebrae. The most frequent presentation is pain and swelling.

Anatomy

Ewing's tumor can be found in soft tissue, as well as bone. Although the disease can occur in any part of the bone, the diaphysis is more commonly involved than the metaphysis. The classical appearance on an x-ray is a diaphyseal tumor with involvement of the medullary cavity (onion-skin appearance), and an associated soft tissue mass.

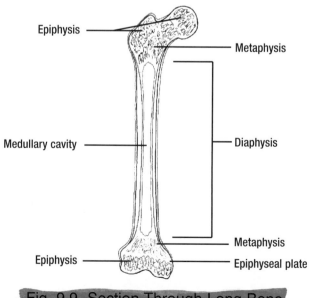

Epiphysis

Metaphysis

Medullary cavity

Diaphysis

Metaphysis

Epiphysis

Epiphyseal plate

Fig. 9.9 Section Through Long Bone

Routes of Spread

Sarcomas most frequently metastasize through the bloodstream. 25% of patients with Ewing's sarcoma will have metastatic disease at diagnosis. The most common metastatic sites are bone or bone marrow, and the lungs. Less than 10% of patients have positive lymph nodes.

Technical Aspects of Radiation Therapy

Multi-drug chemotherapy is indicated in the treatment of all patients because most patients have occult metastatic disease at diagnosis. Local disease is controlled with surgery and/or radiation therapy. Surgery is preferred if the lesion is resectable. Radiation therapy is advocated for patients who do not have a surgical option to preserve function, or to shrink a large tumor preoperatively , or for positive margins after a resection. In patients receiving radiation therapy, strict attention to treatment borders is imperative due to the growing muscles, ligaments and bones in pediatric patients. The target volume is generally the pre-chemotherapy tumor volume from MRI, with at least a 2–3 cm longitudinal margin and a 2 cm lateral margins for long bones. When doses of more than 45 Gy are used, a shrinking field technique may be utilized. Surgical scars and drainage sites must be included in the radiation fields. Bolus may be required. Radiating the entire circumference of the extremity should be avoided to reduce the risk of lymphedema. Growth plates should be avoided in pediatric patients unless they are within the tumor margin, then they should be fully included to avoid asymmetrical growth. Vertebral bodies should either be fully included or spared from the radiation field to prevent uneven height. The Achilles tendon should be excluded whenever possible to prevent late fibrosis after radiation.

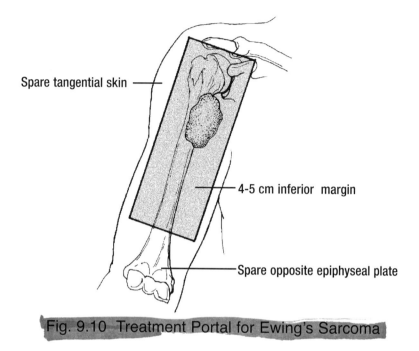

Spare tangential skin

4-5 cm inferior margin

Spare opposite epiphyseal plate

Fig. 9.10 Treatment Portal for Ewing's Sarcoma

Dose

These patients should be entered on protocol when possible. Pre-operative doses of 45-50 Gy may be utilized to shrink the tumor. The definitive radiation dose is typically 55.8 at 1.8 Gy per fraction to the pre-chemotherapy volume.

WILMS' TUMOR

Wilms' tumor, a malignant embryonal tumor of the kidney, is the most common malignant lesion of the genitourinary tract in children. It is bilateral in 5% of the cases. Wilms' tumor predominates in children less than five years of age and is associated with congenital conditions including aniridia, hemihypertrophy and genitourinary abnormalities. Wilms' tumors are divided into favorable and unfavorable histologies. The unfavorable histologies include anaplastic, sarcomatoid, clear cell or rhabdoid features.

Anatomy

Wilms' tumor originates in the kidney. The kidneys are located in the retroperitoneal space. The right kidney is generally 1-2 cm lower than the left because of the position of the liver. Radiographically, the kidneys are located between the 11th rib and the transverse process of L3. The renal axis is parallel to the lateral margin of the psoas muscle.

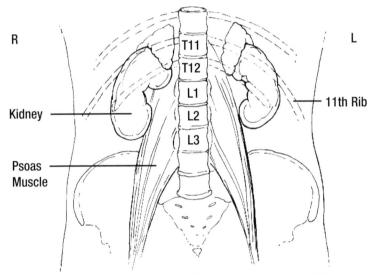

Fig. 9.11   Anatomical Relations of the Kidneys

Routes of Spread

Wilms' tumor may spread through local invasion, lymphatic, or hematogenous routes. The most common sites for distant metastases are the lungs and the liver. Spread through the peritoneal cavity can occur if there is rupture at surgery. Rhabdoid tumors are associated with brain metastases and clear cell sarcoma may metastasize to bone or brain.

Technical Aspects of Radiation Therapy

Surgery is the initial definitive treatment in most cases of Wilms' tumor. All patients then receive systemic chemotherapy. Postoperative radiation to the involved flank is currently recommended in the following cases:

1) All cases of unfavorable histology (Stage I completely resected) excluding anaplastic tumors.
2) Unfavorable histology Stage II (microscopic residual disease)
3) Favorable and unfavorable histology, Stage III (macroscopic residual disease confined to the flank or positive lymph nodes)

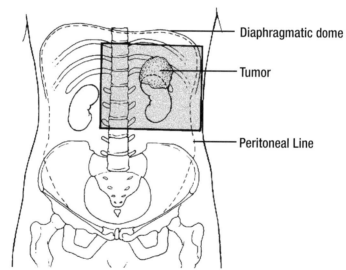

Fig. 9.12 Preoperative Treatment Field for Wilms' Tumor

Lateral: outside peritoneal line
Superior: kidney and entire preoperative tumor extent and 1 cm margin (the field should extend to the dome of the diaphragm only in those patients whose tumor extends to that height)

Medial: lateral to include entire vertebral body to minimize kyphoscoliosis and to include the paraortics (do not overlap contralateral kidney)

Inferior: kidney and entire preoperative tumor extent and 1 cm margin

If peritoneal seeding, diffuse spillage at surgery or pre-operative intraperitoneal rupture is present whole abdomen radiation may be used.

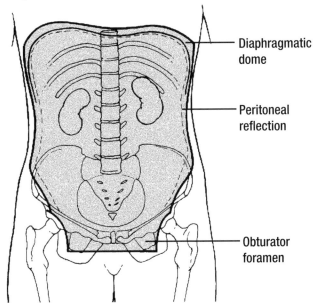

Diaphragmatic dome

Peritoneal reflection

Obturator foramen

Fig. 9.13   Whole Abdomen Treatment Field

Superior: diaphragmatic domes
Lateral: outside peritoneal lines
Inferior: bottom of obturator foramina
(excluding femoral heads and acetabulum)

Dose

A greater than ten day delay of initiation of radiation after surgery has an increased chance of abdominal relapse. For favorable histologies, 10.8 Gy is given at 1.8 Gy/fraction. Boosts are given to "bulk" disease (tumor 3 cm in diameter) including gross disease and 1 cm margin for an additional 10.8 Gy at 1.8 Gy/fraction. The dose to the opposite kidney should be less than 14.4 Gy and no more than one half of the liver should receive 19.8 Gy.

For anaplastic tumors a dose graduate scale is used, depending on the patient age, doses range from 12.6-37.8 Gy.

For whole abdominal treatment 10-12 Gy may be given for favorable histologies, with higher doses for unfavorable histologies. A boost dose to macroscopic residual sites is recommended to a total dose of 20-27 Gy, keeping in mind liver and kidney tolerance. In Stage IV patients with lung involvement, the entire pleural cavity is treated 10.5-15 Gy at 1.5 Gy/fraction with a boost to 20-24 Gy. The abdomen is treated according to operative abdominal stage.

There is a trend in a reduction in treatment volumes and doses to reduce long term side effects. Current protocols must be consulted.

Chapter 10

Soft Tissue Sarcomas

Soft tissue sarcomas are rare, and comprise less than one percent of all cancers. The most common presention is a painless lump or mass. These tumors can grow to a large size, especially in the buttock or thigh, before being diagnosed.

Anatomy

Soft tissue sarcomas arise from the extraskeletal connective tissues of the body (which include the muscles, tendons, fat, fibrous, and synovial tissues). Although they can originate anywhere in the body, approximately 60% will arise in the extremities. For this reason, we will limit our discussion primarily to extremity lesions.

Routes of Spread

Soft tissue sarcomas extend locally and spread along paths of least resistance. Fascial boundaries generally confine the tumor, forming a "pseudo" capsule. Hematogenous spread is common, especially with high grade lesions. The lungs are the most common site of metastasis, and are involved in 50% of the cases. Lymphatics are rarely involved in extremity sarcomas, except in the case of rhabdomyosarcomas, synovial cell sarcomas, or epitheloid sarcomas. The grade of the tumor is the most important prognostic factor in soft tissue sarcomas, and is a predictor of both overall and disease-free survival.

Technical Aspects of Radiation Therapy

Radical surgery, including amputation, has been the treatment of choice for soft tissue sarcomas. In recent years, radiation therapy has proven to be an effective surgical adjunct. When radiation therapy is utilized, less radical surgery is performed, and limbs can often be spared with successful disease control. Both preoperative and postoperative radiation have been used effectively. Advantages of each are listed below:

Post-op Advantages:

-Entire surgical specimen is available for histopathologic review
-Extent of microscopic tumor can be defined
-The surgeon does not have to operate in a previously irradiated tumor bed

Pre-op Advantages

-Allows for shrinkage of the tumor and a less radical operation
-May damage tumor cells on the periphery and prevent dissemination or spread of tumor in the operative site
-Treatment portals are usually smaller
-Pre-op doses are usually less
Treatment planning and careful limb positioning is imperative in the treatment of soft tissue sarcomas. The oncologist must define the muscle and compartment involved, as well as the extent of the lesion based on physical exam, CT, and MRI scans. The exact field margins, proximal and distal to the tumor bed, are controversial. Most oncologists plan a minimum of 5 cm proximal and distal to the tumor bed for low grade lesions, and up to 10 cm for high grade lesions. The entire transverse extent of

the compartment is generally included. Particular attention should be given to sparing a longitudinal strip of normal extremity tissue to decrease the complications of treating the entire cicumference of an extremity. Immobilization of the extremity is important. Low energy photons of 6 MV are recommended for adequate dosing of superficial tissues. The entire superficial scar must be treated and bolus is used if the beam is not tangential to the scar. Regional nodal irradiation is rarely used except with rhabdomyosarcoma, synovial cell sarcomas, or epitheloid sarcomas. In appropriate cases, Intensity Modulated Radiation Therapy (IMRT) may be used to spare critical structures while delivering the prescribed dose to the tumor bed.

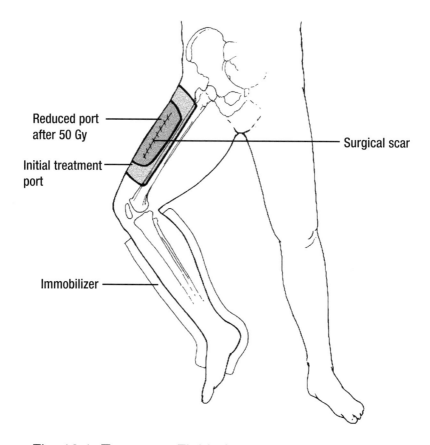

Fig. 10.1 Treatment Fields for Anterior Thigh Sarcoma

Doses

Pre-op doses of 50 Gy with 1.8-2.0 Gy fractions are generally used to the entire treatment volume. Total doses of 60-70 Gy with field reductions at 45-50 Gy and 55-60 Gy are generally employed post-operatively.

Interstitial brachytherapy may be utilized as a boost following pre-op external beam and surgery.

Chapter 11

Emergencies

Emergent treatment is required for tumors that involve the spinal canal and result in spinal cord compression. Treatment should be initiated immediately to reduce the risk of permanent neurological damage.

Tumors that infiltrate the mediastinum and compress the superior vena cava can cause life-threatening complications. Immediate therapy is indicated to alleviate brain edema, reduced cardiac output or upper airway obstruction.

For both spinal cord compression and superior vena cava syndrome, it is generally recommended that treatment be started within several hours of the time of diagnosis, when the symptoms are minimal.

SPINAL CORD COMPRESSION

Compression of the spinal cord is most commonly caused by metastasis to the spine. Tumors most commonly extend posteriorly through the bony canal into the space around the spinal cord (epidural space). The four most common presenting symptoms of spinal cord compression include: pain, weakness, autonomic dysfunction (loss of bowel and bladder sphincter control), and sensory loss. Carcinoma of the lung, prostate, breast, and lymphomas are the most common primary tumors that may cause spinal cord compression.

Diagnosis of possible spinal cord compression can be made following careful neurologic exam, CT or MRI.

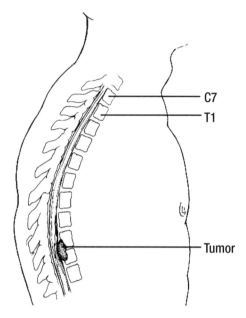

Fig. 11.1 Compression on Mid-Thoracic Spinal Cord

Treatment

The use of corticosteroids and radiation therapy play important roles in the treatment of spinal cord compression. Once the diagnosis of cord compression has been made, high doses of dexamethasone are recommended. Surgery is indicated when there has been no histologic diagnosis of cancer, or when x-rays demonstrate a collapsed vertebra. Under these circumstances, emergency laminectomy followed by postoperative radiation is recommended. Surgery is also indicated when there is evidence of recurrent cancer and the spinal cord has previously reached radiation tolerance.

Technical Aspects of Radiation Therapy

Following the administration of corticosteroids, external beam radiation is the treatment of choice for most patients. Imaging studies are used to determine the upper and lower extent of tumor involvement. Generally, a 3-4 cm margin is placed above and below the lesion. Many oncologists prefer a margin of two vertebral bodies above and below the cord compression.

Treatment Borders for a Spinal Cord Compression:

Superior: 3-4 cm above the cord compression
Inferior: 3-4 cm below the cord compression
Lateral: Typically 7-8 cm wide, but may vary according to the lateral extent of the tumor.

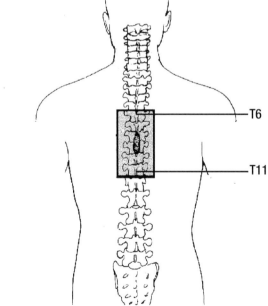

Fig. 11.2 Spinal Cord Compression Port

Dose

The dose schedule may vary but typical total doses range from 30-40 Gy in two to four weeks. The initial fractionation schedule should be higher (3.5-4.0 Gy per fraction), for three to four treatments in an attempt to maximize the response as soon as possible. Doses as high as 8 Gy in a single fraction have been used for 1-2 fractions for patients with a short-term prognosis.

SUPERIOR VENA CAVA SYNDROME

Obstruction of the superior vena cava by a mediastinal mass produces a medical emergency requiring immediate treatment. The superior vena cava represents the major venous channel for return of blood to the heart from the upper thorax, head, neck and upper extremities. Anatomically, the superior vena cava is surrounded by the anterior mediastinal structures and encircled by numerous lymph nodes.

The two most common malignant causes of the syndrome are lung cancer and lymphomas, accounting for 90-95% of all cases. Benign conditions of the syndrome, such as thyroid goiter, account for only 2-3% of cases. The most common presenting symptoms of superior vena cava syndrome are shortness of breath, facial swelling, distension of the veins of the neck and thorax, chest pain, cough, and dysphagia.

A CT scan of the chest will usually determine the location of the tumor. Obstruction of the superior vena cava may occur secondary to extensive compression by tumor or lymph nodes, or by direct invasion of tumor into the vessel wall, with or without associated thrombosis.

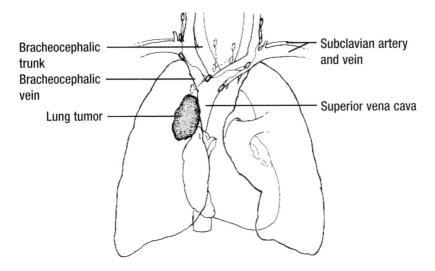

Bracheocephalic trunk

Bracheocephalic vein

Lung tumor

Subclavian artery and vein

Superior vena cava

Fig. 11.3 Superior Vena Cava Compression by Lung Tumor

Treatment

Initiation of treatment should be immediate for patients who are symptomatic, even though a tissue diagnosis has not been established. Once the symptoms have been relieved and the patient is clinically stable (possibly following only three to four radiation treatments), a thorough work-up and diagnosis, including biopsy can be performed safely.

External beam radiation therapy is initiated as soon as possible and is considered the treatment of choice. Chemotherapy may be given initially for patients diagnosed with small cell carcinoma of the lung, who present with superior vena cava syndrome. Many oncologists advocate the addition of steroids, especially in cases of acute respiratory compromise. Anticoagulants may also be used, especially if thrombosis is suspected and there has been limited response to radiation therapy.

Technical Aspects of Radiation Therapy

In cases with full blown superior vena cava syndrome and
respiratory compromise, the patient may require treatment
on a slant board to elevate the chest and head. The
treatment portal should include the primary tumor with a
2-3 cm margin, and the mediastinal, hilar and
supraclavicular areas.

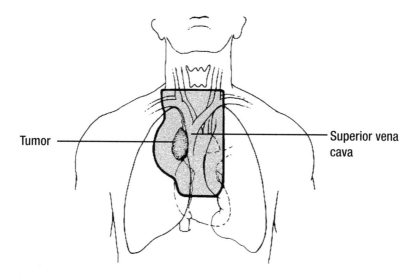

Tumor —   — Superior vena
cava

Fig. 11.4 Treatment Field for Superior Vena Cava Syndrome

Dose

Initially several high fractions (3-4 Gy) are given for two to
four days followed by conventional fractionation of 1.5-2.0
Gy daily. Total doses depend on the exact histology of the
tumor.

REFERENCES

Ang K. K., Kaanders J., Peters L., (Eds). (1994). Radiotherapy for head and neck cancers: indications and techniques, Philadelphia, PA: Lea & Febiger.

Auberdiac P, Charqari C., Negrier F., Boutinaud C., Zioueche A., Cartier L., ... Magne N. (2012). Magnetic resonance imaging for delineation of prostate in radiotherapy: monocentric experience and review of literature. *Prog Urol* 22(3), 159-165.

Bentel C.(1995). Radiation Therapy Planning. 2nd ed. New York, NY: McGraw-Hill Inc.

Bentel G., Nelson C., Noell K. (1989). Treatment Planning and Dose Calculation in Radiation Oncology. 4 th Edition. Pergamon Press.

Caglar H., Allen A., Othus M., Li Y., Burke E., Wirth L., et al. (2008). Dose to the larynx predicts for swallowing complications following IMRT and chemotherapy. *Int J Radiat Oncol Biol Phys* 72(4),1110-1118.

Chao K Clifford (2005). Practical Essentials of Intensity Modulated Radiation Therapy, 2nd ed. Philadelphia, PA: Lippincott Williams & Wilkins.

Clemente C. (2007). Anatomy: A Regional Atlas of the Human Body. 5th ed. Philadelphia, PA: Lippincott Williams & Wilkins.

Cox J. Moss' Radiation Oncology: Rationale, Techniques, Results. 7th ed. St. Louis, MO: Mosby-Year Book Inc; 1994.

D'Angio G., Sinniah D., Meadows A., Evans A., Pritchard J. (Eds.). (1992). Practical Pediatric Oncology. London: Edward Arnold Co.

DeVita Jr., V., Hellman S., Rosenberg S., (Eds.). (2011). Cancer: Principles & Practice of Oncology. 9th ed. Philadelphia, PA: Lippincott Williams and Wilkins.

Fleckenstein P., Tranum-Jensen, J. (2001). Anatomy in Diagnostic Imaging. 2nd ed. Philadelphia, PA: W.B. Saunders Company.

Fletcher G. (1980). Textbook of Radiotherapy (Ed. 3). Philadelphia, PA, Lea & Febiger.

Goodman K. (2012) Anal and rectal cancers: anatomy, contouring and considerations for IMRT planning (PDF document). Retrieved January 20, 2013 from: http://www.astro.org

Grégoire V., De Neve W., Eisbruch A., Lee N., Van Den Weyngaert D. & Van Gestelin D. (2007). Intensity-modulated radiation therapy for head and neck carcinoma. The Oncologist.

Halperin E. (1998). Pediatric Radiation Oncology. 3rd ed. Philadelphia, PA: Lippincott Williams & Wilkins Publishers.

Halperin E., Perez C., Brady L. (Eds). (2008). Principles and Practice of Radiation Oncology. 5th ed. Philadelphia, Pa: Lippincott Williams & Wilkins.

Harris J., Hellman S., Henderson I., Kinne D. (Eds). (1991). Breast diseases. 2nd ed. Philadelphia : JB Lippincott Company.

Holleb A., Fink D., Murphy G. (1991). Textbook of Clinical Oncology. Atlanta, Ga: American Cancer Society.

International Commission on Radiation Units and Measurements. (1993). ICRU Report 50. Prescribing, recording, and reporting photon beam therapy. Bethesda, MD.

International Commission on Radiation Units and Measurements. (1999). ICRU Report 62. Prescribing, recording, and reporting photon beam therapy (Supplement to ICRU Report 50). Bethesda, MD.

Jagsi R., Moran D., Marsh R., Masi K., Griffith K. & Pierce L. (2010). Evaluation of four techniques using intensity-modulated radiation therapy for comprehensive locoregional irradiation of breast cancer. *Int J Radiat Oncol Biol Phys, 78(5)*, 1594-1603.

Kehwar T.S., Sharma S.C. (2003). Use of normal tissue tolerance doses into linear quadratic equation to estimate normal tissue complication probability. *Radiat Oncol Online J.* Retrieved October 13, 2012 from: http://www.rooj.com

Levitt J., Seymour H., et al, (Eds). (2006). Technological Basis of Radiation Therapy: Practical Clinical Applications. 4th ed. Berlin, N.Y.: Springer.

Milosevic M., Voruganti S., Blend R., Alasti H., Warde P., McLean M., ... Gospodarowicz M. (1998). Magnetic resonance imaging (MRI) for localization of the prostatic apex: comparison to computed tomography (CT) and urethrography. *Radiotherapy and Oncology, 47(3)*, 277-284.

Myerson R., Garofalo M., El Naqa I., Abrams R., Apte A., Bosch W., Das P., ...Kachnic L. (2009). Elective clinical target volumes for conformal therapy in anorectal cancer: a radiation therapy oncology group consensus panel contouring atlas. *Int J Radiat Oncol Biol Phys* 74(3), 824-830.

Myrehaug S, Chan G, Craig T, Weinberg V, Cheng C, Roach M 3rd, Cheung P, Sahgal A. (2012). A treatment planning and acute toxicity comparison of two pelvic nodal volume delineation techniques and delivery comparison of intensity-modulated radiotherapy versus volumetric modulated arc therapy for hypofractionated high-risk prostate cancer radiotherapy. *Int J Radiat Oncol Biol Phys* 82(4) 657-662.

National Cancer Institute. Late Effects of Treatment for Childhood Cancer. Retrieved March 26, 2013 from: http://www.cancer.gov/cancertopics/pdq/treatment/lateeff ects/HealthProfessional.

National Cancer Institute (NCI). The National Cancer Institute Guidelines for the Use of Intensity-Modulated Radiation Therapy in Clinical Trials. Bethesda, MD: NCI; July 24, 2012. Retrieved September 25, 2012 from: http://atc.wustl.edu/home/NCI/IMRT_NCI_Guidelines_v4. 0.pdf

National Cancer Institute. Childhood acute lymphoblastic leukemia treatment. Retrieved March 26, 2013 from: http://www.cancer.gov/cancertopics/pdq/treatment/childA LL/Patient/page4.

National Cancer Institute. Wilms' Tumor and other Childhood Kidney Tumors Treatment. Retrieved March 26, 2013 from: http://www.cancer.gov/cancertopics/pdq/treatment/wilms /HealthProfessional.

Netter F. (1989). Atlas of Human Anatomy. Summit, NJ: CIBA-GEIGY.

Packer R.J., Allen J.C., Goldwein J.L., Newall J., Zimmerman R.A., Priest J., ...D'Angio G. (1990). Hyperfactionated radiotherapy for children with brainstem gliomas: a pilot study using 7,200cGy. *Annals of Neurology* 27(2), 167-173.

Pejavar S., Polley M.Y., Rosenberg-Wohl S., Chennupati S., Prados M.D., Berger M.S., ...Haas-Kogan D. (2012). Pediatric intracranial ependymoma: the roles of surgery, radiation and chemotherapy. *J Neurooncol* 106(2), 367-375.

Perez C., Brady L. (1997). Principles & Practices of Radiation Oncology. 3rd ed. Philadelphia, PA: Lippincott-Raven Publishing.

Reshma J., Phil D., Moran J., Marsh R., Masi K., Griffith K., Pierce L. (2010). Evaluation of four techniques using intensity-modulated radiation therapy for comprehensive locoregional irradiation of breast cancer. *Int J Radiat Oncol Biol Phy* 78(5), 1594-1603.

Vieillot S., Azria D., Lemanski C., Moscardo C.L., Gourgou S., Dubois J., ...Fenoglietto P. (2010). Plan comparison of volumetric-modulated arc therapy (RapidArc) and conventional intensity-modulated radiation therapy (IMRT) in anal canal cancer. *Radiation Oncology* 5(1) 92-99.

Stryker J. (1992). Clinical Oncology for Students of Radiation Therapy Technology. St. Louis, MO, Warren H. Green Inc.

Spalding A., Kyung W., Vineberg K., Jablonowsk M., Fraass B., Pan C., ... Ben-Josef E. (2007). Potential for dose-escalation and reduction of risk in pancreatic cancer using IMRT optimization with lexicographic ordering and geud-based cost functions. *Medical Physics* 34(2), 521-529.

Urbano M. T., Henrys A.J., Adams E.J., Norman A.R., Bedford J.L., Harrington K.J., ...Tait D.M. (2006). Intensity-modulated radiotherapy in patients with locally advanced rectal cancer reduces volume of bowel treated to high dose levels. *Int J Radiat Oncol Biol Phys* 65(3), 907-916.

Wang C. (1997). Radiation Therapy for Head and Neck Neoplasms. 4th ed. New York, NY: Wiley-Liss, Inc.

Welsh J., Palmer M., Ajani J., Liao Z., Sweisher S., Hofstetter W., ...Komaki R. (2012). Esophageal cancer dose escalation using a simultaneous integrated boost technique. *Int J Radiat Oncol Biol Phys* 82(1), 468-474.

Radiation Therapy: Hodgkin's Lymphoma Health Guide. The New York Times. Retrieved September 10, 2012 from: http://health.nytimes.com

Yap J., Malhotra H., Yang G. (2010). Intensity modulated radiation therapy in the treatment of esophageal cancer. *Thoracic Cancer* 1, 62-69.

(1990). Errata. *Journal of Clinical Oncology*, Vol 8 (9), 1602. Retrieved September 10, 2012 from: http://jco.ascopubs.org